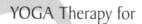

YOGA Therapy for

Overcoming Insomnia

YOGA Therapy for

Overcoming Insomnia

Peter Van Houten, M.D., and Gyandev Rich McCord, Ph.D.

Crystal Clarity Publishers
Nevada City, California

Design by Crystal Clarity Publishers
Photography by Sugar Pine Studios
Illustrations by Karen White

ISBN: 1-56589-174-0
Printed in China
3 5 7 9 10 8 6 4 2

Crystal Clarity Publishers
14618 Tyler Foote Road
Nevada City, CA 95959-8599

800.424.1055 OR 530.478.7600
fax: 530.478.7610
clarity@crystalclarity.com
www.crystalclarity.com

Library of Congress Cataloging-in-Publication Data
Van Houten, Peter.
  Yoga therapy for overcoming insomnia / Peter Van Houten and Gyandev McCord.
     p. cm.
  Includes bibliographical references and index.
  ISBN 1-56589-174-0 (hbk. : alk. paper)
  1. Insomnia—Alternative treatment. 2. Hatha yoga—Therapeutic use. I. McCord, Rich. II. Title.
  RC548.V355 2004
  616.8'498206—dc22   2004022559

Table of Contents

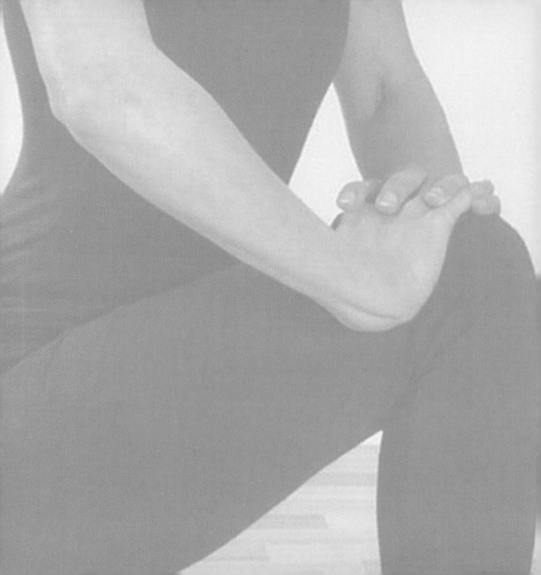

Introduction

"Doc, if I could just get a good night's sleep…"

You look at your bedside clock and it's 3:00AM and you think, "Oh no, not another night when I don't sleep! I have so much to do tomorrow!" If this is happening to you, there is help available right now. You are not alone with the problem of insomnia. Roughly half the adults in our culture have some trouble with insomnia, and some have a severe, debilitating form of it. Whether your insomnia is mild and occasional or an every night torture, this book can help you. Using the latest scientific research, we will give you a clear understanding of the nature of insomnia, including its common causes and treatments. This is a comprehensive program that you can start using tonight for deep, sound sleep.

As a cornerstone of our treatment plan, we will be using the well-known Ananda Yoga™ system as a way to let you relax deeply and prepare your mind and body for refreshing sleep. You'll learn how you can deeply relax at will using specific yoga postures, stretches, methods of relaxation, breathing techniques, and affirmations.

These techniques, when performed along with our recommendations for healthy sleep habits, can give you the sound sleep you are wanting. You can work with this program on your own, or you can use this approach in conjunction with any treatment your physician recommends. The healthy sleep habits suggested in this book are ones that most physicians wholeheartedly endorse. Your health care provider may have already recommended this book or activities like this.

You'll find that most physicians are already familiar with the positive effects that relaxation, affirmation, attitude, habit changes, and stretching techniques can have on a host of medical problems, including insomnia. For example, one study done on insomnia in 2001 demonstrated that simply modifying a person's attitudes about sleep and teaching them good sleep habits produced better long-term outcomes than giving them medication! The great news is that most people can be taught routines for ensuring sound sleep that will be effective for a lifetime.

You'll find this is an excellent handbook with enjoyable, and highly effective, yoga routines and other sleep recommendations that you can start using today. Help is on the way. Get ready for a great night's sleep!

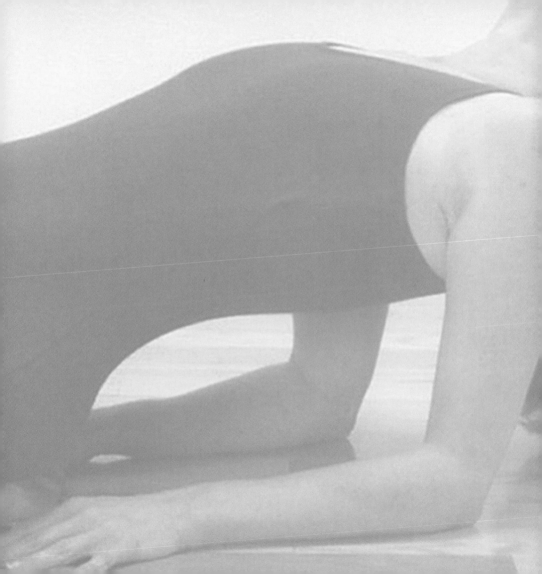

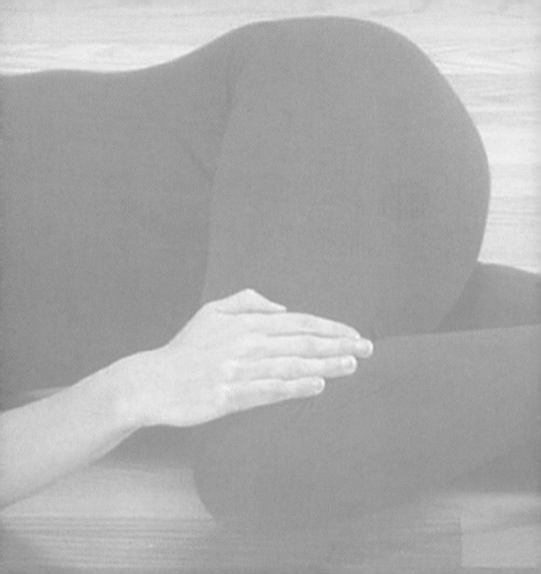

A Note on the
Yoga Practices in This Book

This book is designed to blend seamlessly with the medical care you may already be receiving for insomnia. Any actual changes in your medication or treatment should, of course, be made in consultation with your health care provider.

While the exercises we present here are simple, not all yoga practices are suitable for everyone. To reduce the risk of injury, it's a good idea to consult your doctor before beginning any exercise program like this one. Obviously, the instructions and advice in this book are not intended as substitutes for medical counsel from your health care advisor. At the end of Chapter Nine, we offer specific recommendations for those few who do not find adequate improvement after trying the suggestions in this book.

The therapeutic approach in this book is intended to benefit a wide range of people suffering from insomnia, and for most people it is an excellent starting point. To get the greatest therapeutic benefit, it's even better to work individually with a qualified yoga instructor who can draw upon a broader range of yoga therapy techniques and tailor your program to your unique needs and abilities. Bear in mind that although yoga therapy often may improve insomnia symptoms immediately, usually it is not a "quick fix" like a sleeping pill. It is a gradual route to creating lasting harmony on all levels of your being.

There are many common medical problems like insomnia that either have ineffective medical treatments or have treatments that are effective but require expensive or side effect laden pharmaceutical medications. For example, roughly ten percent of adults in the U.S. have chronic nightly insomnia problems and are faced with the reality that the best medications for insomnia can cost $3 a pill and are habit forming. Twenty percent of adults in the U.S. are uninsured and many others "underinsured," lacking any meaningful medication coverage. Obviously, there is a need for safe and inexpensive, non-drug, "behavioral" treatments that are easy to teach. In fact, behavioral treatments are desperately needed for many medical conditions, not just insomnia. Unfortunately, most physicians don't have the time or the training to teach behavioral solutions to their patients, particularly when it is so quick and easy to reach for the prescription pad.

In addition, in medicine today, any treatment a physician recommends should be "evidence based." That is, there must be scientific studies showing that a medication or behavioral treatment has actually been shown to work in controlled studies. Fortunately, there is solid science supporting relaxation techniques, affirmations, stretching exercises, and breathing exercises for treating insomnia. The dilemma most physicians and their patients find is that most of the typically recommended behavioral techniques for insomnia are pretty uninteresting and dull for the patient. As you might expect, the dropout rate among patients is, therefore, often high. Some of the main reasons we chose Ananda Yoga as a treatment tool are that it is well known with certified teachers, it emphasizes relaxation, it can incorporate breathing exercises, it uses "self talk" affirmations, and it uses gentle yoga stretches. Here is a program that is easy to do and has multiple evidence-based components. AND, best of all, it is actually fun for someone to do. Clearly a person is much more likely to continue with something that is part of a unified program and is enjoyable. After reading this book, if you would like more information about Ananda Yoga and actual personal instruction, see Chapter Eleven: Next Steps with Ananda Yoga.

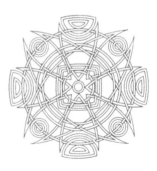

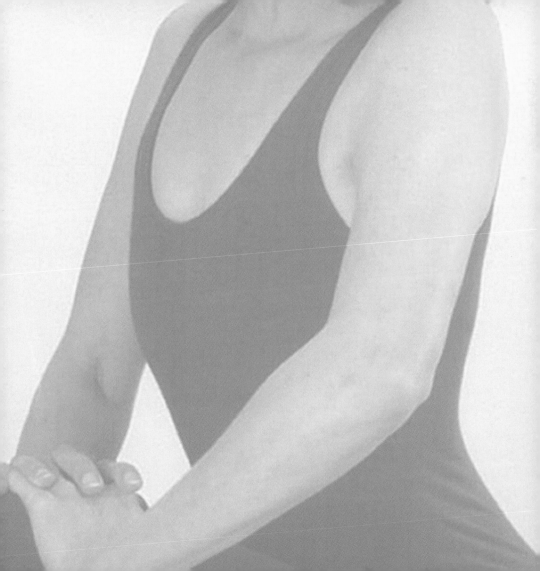

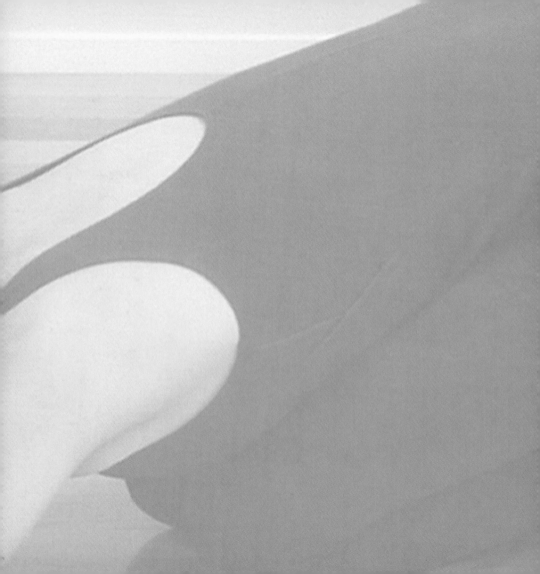

Chapter One

✳

Insomnia Is a Major Problem

Almost everyone has an occasional problem with sleeping poorly. It may be the night before a final exam in school or during a time of major stress, such as the death of a loved one. Many people have experienced the insomnia associated with severe jet lag after a long airline trip. You know how frustrating it can be to be unable to sleep when you want to, but your body wants to be wide awake! In fact, close to 50% of people in our culture have an intermittent but recurrent problem with difficulty sleeping. Insomnia is the most common disorder of sleep. It's also one of the most frequent reasons a person visits a doctor. While for most insomnia is just occasional, for some it is a chronic problem of nightly insomnia that pesters them for months or years. About 10% of people have some ongoing insomnia *nightly*—a huge number, particularly when you consider how debilitating insomnia can be.

Case Study #1—Mike:
He Just Can't Fall Asleep

Mike recently graduated from college and now has a responsible job with an accounting firm. He often has to take work home to complete in the evening but is expected to be at work ready to go at 8am the next day. He enjoys his work but just wishes he could stop thinking about all the details when he's done for the day. About three months ago, he began having some problems falling asleep—not every night—but about half the time. Typically, once he fell asleep, he slept pretty soundly. However, this last month he's had trouble falling asleep every single night.

Once he didn't fall asleep until an hour before his alarm went off and he felt really awful the next day! He's never had a sleep problem before.

Everyone has suggestions for him about his insomnia. He's tried doing a really hot bath and an aerobics workout just before bed so he'd be really tired and relaxed but, amazingly, it just made him more awake than ever. One friend recommended a stiff drink of brandy every night as cure, while others have suggested their favorite bedtime herbal remedy. So far he's tried every single suggestion. Some even help for a few nights before they stop working. Mike is actually starting to get nervous when he knows bedtime is approaching. Mike thinks to himself, "Not another night where I can't go to sleep! I just can't stand it." The quality of his work has begun slipping, and he's getting grouchy and irritable. Once he even slept right through his alarm and was three hours late for work. He sees prescription sleep medication advertised everywhere, but he doesn't want to get addicted to a medication. Mike sees that his insomnia problem is now a downward spiral, but he hasn't got a clue what to do.

It turns out that Mike's particular insomnia problem is likely straightforward and common. Simply put, he has developed very poor sleep "habits," and his body and mind have learned this insomnia behavior very well in just a few short months! Fortunately for Mike, he can easily learn the right habits and attitudes for sound sleep. When this is coupled with special relaxation techniques to get him ready for sleep every night, his problem will likely vanish within weeks. Also, he'll have a clear understanding of how to keep his sleep deep and refreshing for a lifetime. The techniques and information in this book would be ideal for him.

Susan is a high school teacher who loves teaching. About six months ago, her marriage of eight years ended. Even though she and her "ex" parted on friendly terms she's been feeling pretty flat emotionally and nothing seems to interest her much. For example, she hasn't had her normal energy for preparing lesson plans for school. Right after the break-up, she began having sleep problems. She falls asleep without difficulty—in fact, she looks forward to going to bed, hoping tomorrow she'll be rested and energetic. But after a few hours she wakes up and can't go back to sleep—usually for about an hour but sometimes for the rest of the night! She keeps waking up every few hours until morning. On school days, she wishes she could "sleep in" but she needs to get up and get ready for work. Sometimes on the weekend she'll stay in bed for 14 hours at a stretch but will actually sleep only about half of that—the rest of the time she just lies there. She had trouble like this about fifteen years ago after she lost her job during a "downsizing" at her previous school. That time, however, her sleep got better after a few months.

Now she's stopped exercising simply because she's too tired in the evening, and she's gained about ten pounds in the last three months. She stopped seeing friends in the evening because she wants to get to bed early. Her self-esteem is in the dumps. She finally went to her doctor to get some sleeping pills and, to her surprise, was offered an anti-depressant medication. She told her doctor, "I'm not depressed. In fact, if I just had a good night's sleep, I'd be fine. I just need a pill to keep me asleep."

Susan has a kind of insomnia sometimes called "early awakening," where she awakens in the middle of the night and can't go back to sleep. Susan's insomnia is probably caused by the mild depression she's experiencing. Her sleep disturbance is actually one of the symptoms that are clues to her depression. While for most people insomnia is simply a sleep disorder, for some it is the chief sign of an underlying problem like depression or anxiety. Susan also made her insomnia symptoms worse by some of the negative lifestyle changes she's recently made, like stopping her exercise program. Susan will benefit from a sleep program such as the one outlined in this book, but she may need to address her depression more directly if her symptoms continue.

What is Insomnia?

Simply put, insomnia is the inability to have a refreshing night's sleep when you want it. The problems that are typical in insomnia include difficulty falling asleep or waking up during the night and being unable to return to sleep rapidly, as we've seen in our two case studies. The key to understanding insomnia is that it's not about the total amount of sleep time one has, it's the inability to have sleep that leaves one refreshed in the morning. Sleep requirements are actually highly individual. One person may feel completely recharged after only six hours sleep. Another may require a full eight hours for the same level of rejuvenation. If you are an "eight-hour-a-night" person who sleeps only six hours, you may feel sleep deprived the next day.

Not everyone who gets inadequate sleep is suffering from insomnia. Many people who are sleep deprived are missing sleep by choice or because they are forced by their circumstances to limit their sleep time. For example, a surgeon on night call at a hospital or a mother caring for her sick children may get less than three hours of sleep one night, which is enough to hurt their function the next day. However, they may not have any problem with insomnia. Given the chance to sleep, and they would probably love it, they will sleep normally.

The Consequences of Inadequate Sleep

Sleep deprivation caused by insomnia or by simply not sleeping enough can affect your daytime function tremendously. If you are sleep deprived, you can have memory problems, difficulty concentrating, poor social interactions, daytime sleepiness and fatigue, as well as annoying symptoms of physical stress such as headaches and gastrointestinal woes. There are even problems with decreased immune function. While those with mild or short-term insomnia (less than a month) may find this has limited effects on their daytime function, those with chronic insomnia may have significant trouble with their performance during the day. For example, those with chronic insomnia are twice as likely to have auto accidents as those who sleep normally.

Many people in our culture are not sleeping enough. Students often stay up late but leave for school very early, and some are chronically under-sleeping. People who work at jobs that have "shifts" may sleep less. Because they sleep and work at unusual times compared to the rest of us, the typical shift worker sleeps eight hours less a week than those with normal work schedules. Some professions, such as health care, demand long hours of night call with little or no sleep. Our culture as a whole sleeps 25% less than our ancestors did a hundred years ago, but there is no evidence that we need less sleep than they did. Also, with the current 24-hour-a-day availability of TV, shopping, and the Internet, we can find many excuses at home to delay or forgo adequate sleep.

When a person's sleep patterns become distorted by choice or life's circumstances, they may go on to develop insomnia and not be able to sleep when they want to. This very common form of insomnia is actually from bad sleep habits their bodies have learned. This was Mike's problem in our case studies. Poor sleep habits are often referred to as "poor sleep hygiene."

It Can Be Hard to Tell How Sleep Deprivation Is Affecting You

Those who are sleep deprived may be unaware how impaired they are. One study done at a sleep laboratory where volunteers were kept awake constantly for days at a time found that the mental abilities of the subjects, as measured by standardized tests, worsened with each passing day. The curious thing was that the volunteers often commented that, as the number of sleepless days increased, they felt they were "adjusting to the lack of sleep" and were convinced they were starting to perform better on those tests, even as their actual scores worsened!

Studies on sleep deprived professional truck drivers, done in a laboratory using driving sim-ulators, found that they often couldn't tell they were beginning to nod off while driving. They would simply awake with great surprise to find they had driven the simulator "into a ditch!"

One sobering study looked at how surgeons performed the day after spending a night on call when they got less than three hours total sleep. They were compared to surgeons who were normally rested when performing a particular surgical task. The "under-slept" surgeons took 40% longer doing the surgical task and made twice as many errors—all from just one night of very inadequate sleep! Frequent insomnia can cause significant sleep deprivation over time and potentially put you, and those around you, at risk.

Insomnia:
a 100 Billion Dollar Problem

As you can see, those with insomnia may really be suffering. The less you sleep because of insomnia, the more likely you are to feel lousy and have other sleep deprivation symptoms the following day. With very intermittent insomnia there may be little in the way of bad effects. However, if you have severe chronic insomnia, you are quite likely to have significant impairments and complaints. Roughly half of those with insomnia complain of not feeling well physically, which finally gets them to go see a doctor. Longstanding insomnia predisposes you to depression and anxiety problems. Some people develop tremendous anxiety over not sleeping well, as we saw in Mike's case.

Out of frustration at being unable to sleep, many insomniacs become dependent on alcohol or other sedatives to put them to sleep. In fact, about 10% of alcoholics became alcohol dependent **because** of insomnia initially! Many others take non-prescription sleeping pills nightly, and the side effects of these drugs can also negatively affect their function the next day. You can end up dependent on over-the-counter medications that give only unnatural and unrefreshing sleep.

Put bluntly, the effect of insomnia on our culture is catastrophic. The costs of all the problems caused by insomnia are staggering—particularly if we look at those who are sleeping less than five and a half hours a night. If we include fatigue-related accidents, poor job performance, absenteeism, and the expense of sleep medications, the cost totals over 100 billion dollars a year! There are untold deaths yearly from auto accidents caused by sleepy drivers. Lost jobs, lost promotions, lost friendships, and decreased productivity at work can all result from the simple inability to sleep.

Not Many with Insomnia Seek
Medical Help—and Many Doctors
Have Difficulty Treating Insomnia

Surprisingly few insomniacs, even those with severe symptoms, seek medical help. Less than 15% of those with insomnia have seen a doctor, and less than a third of those seen come away from their visit with a clear understanding of their problem. When a patient with insomnia visits their doctor, they may find their physician is ill equipped to help them. The scientific understanding of insomnia and its treatment has advanced considerably in the last twenty years, but the average physician's understanding has often lagged behind. Even many conscientious physicians don't understand that patients really need to be educated in depth about insomnia and need to be taught about ways they can help themselves to sleep better—not simply given a sleeping pill prescription.

Studies reveal that the treatment of insomnia tends to be frustrating, and frequently unsatisfactory, for both the patient and the doctor. When confronted with a somewhat desperate patient with severe insomnia, the average physician may inwardly be saying, "Oh no, not another one!" Often physicians simply reach for their prescription pads out of frustration or a lack of time. The drugs typically prescribed for insomnia by physicians are designed for short term or occasional use only. No one really wants to be dependent on drugs to sleep.

There is good news, however. Modern research has shown that giving a patient a few simple lifestyle rules, easy and enjoyable techniques to help relax, and specific suggestions for their sleep routine works as well as prescription sleeping pills, *and* it is natural sleep, not chemically induced. These techniques will often provide a lasting "fix" to sleep problems. Even if medication is needed initially as an aid, it can often be discontinued over time as long as you are doing other positive things to keep sleeping well.

Obviously, in the long run helping you change your sleep habits and routine, teaching you relaxation techniques to prepare for sleep, and giving you positive sleep affirmations, is more helpful and much safer than taking sleeping pills. This book will train you to use the Ananda Yoga system as a way of improving your sleep. When done in conjunction with the other well-researched lifestyle modifications we suggest, it is a powerful tool to restore normal sleep patterns. Using this "non-drug" approach to insomnia, the vast majority of people will not only sleep better but many will eliminate their use of sleep medication.

First let's look at what constitutes normal sleep and some of the causes of insomnia. Then we'll show you how Ananda Yoga can be used in a program to improve your sleep patterns. Lastly, we'll look at other practical suggestions for getting a great night's sleep.

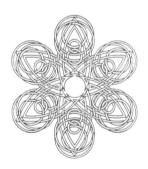

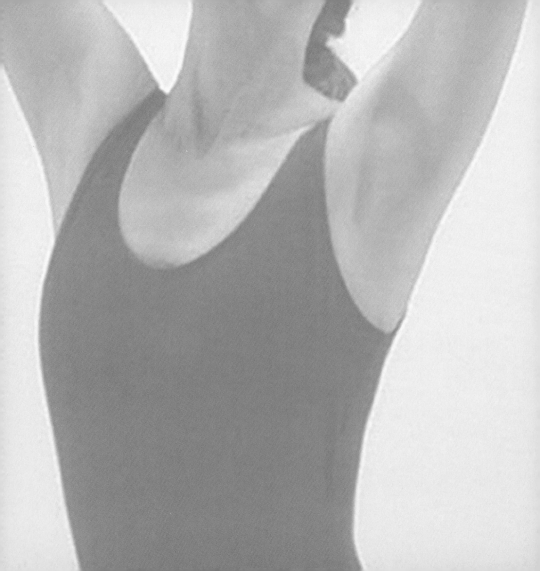

Chapter Two

✴

Everything You Ever Wanted to Know About Sleep

Sleep is an important time of restoration and is critical for both your physical and mental health. During sleep your brain processes memories and information from the day, which is important to learning. Sleep even includes a nightly boost in your immune system's function.

Your brain, primarily through your 24-hour "body clock" or circadian rhythms, controls your sleep patterns. Keeping track of your body clock is one of your brain's many "janitorial" functions. The body clock function of your brain determines your times for sleep and waking. It does this by affecting your body temperature and by the daily release of certain hormones that affect alertness.

Sleep Cycles

During normal sleep we cycle between two main types of sleep:

dream sleep and non-dream sleep. Both types of sleep have specific characteristics that make them easy to distinguish. Dream sleep, which is also referred to as REM (rapid eye movement) sleep, is when your brain is very active and you may experience dreaming. Curiously, despite the increased brain activity, your body is essentially non-moving and your muscles are completely relaxed. Your pulse rate and breathing, however, tend to be increased. Also, your eyes are moving underneath closed eyelids, hence the term rapid eye movement or REM sleep.

The remainder of your sleep time is composed of non-dream or non-REM sleep. Non-REM sleep is a state of deep rest with slowing of your pulse rate and respirations. Your brain's activity is low. In non-REM sleep you typically pass through four stages from light sleep (stage 1) to deep sleep (stages 3 and 4).

Roughly every 90 minutes we go through a full sleep cycle including REM sleep and all four stages of non-REM sleep. Then a new cycle starts. Typically people have four or five of these 90- minute cycles every night. As the night progresses you have more REM, or dream sleep, in each cycle and less non-REM in each 90-minute cycle. You spend about 25% of your total sleep time in REM sleep and about 20% in deep sleep (stage 3 and 4). You will likely notice more dreaming in the hours just before awakening.

How Much Sleep Do You Need?

The amount of sleep you require is highly individual and can vary with your physical and psychological health as well as your stress level. Your baseline average sleep need is mostly an inherited trait. Although some people with normal sleep patterns require less than seven hours a night, most need seven to eight hours of sleep to feel refreshed. The amount of adequate sleep people require ranges from about four to ten hours a night, and this amount is also affected by such factors as your current age. The quality of your sleep gets poorer as you age, with more frequent awakenings and less time spent in deep sleep. You can see why people describe great sleep as "sleeping like a baby!" Fortunately, it's been shown that even elderly people with insomnia will respond well to the therapies we are recommending in this book. No matter what your age, you need to find your own personal minimum amount of sleep, typically between seven and eight hours, that lets you feel refreshed.

Body Temperature
Changes as a Key to Sleep

Your body temperature varies in cycles over a 24-hour period, with the range between high and low being about 1.5 degrees F. Your brain keys on a decline in body temperature as the sign it's time to start sleep. We are most alert when our body temperature is peaking and sleepiest when it is bottoming out. Having a standard bedtime and, even more important, a standard awakening time keeps our body clock in synchrony and our sleep cycles regular. You can see why exercising or taking a very hot bath, both of which raise your body temperature, right before bedtime may interfere with you falling asleep. Your exact body temperature cycles are unique. You've probably noticed that some people are "toast," that is, they pop out of bed ready to go in the morning (like toast popping out of a toaster) and tend to be at their worst at night. Others are "night owls" who seem brightest when others are heading for bed. Toast people tend to have higher than average body temperatures on awakening, while night owls tend to be higher than most just before bed. Interestingly, exposure to light also affects your body temperature cycle and can even be used to reset your cycle!

Melatonin

Sunlight and darkness also affect our sleep times through the brain's production of melatonin, which is a natural sleep-inducing brain chemical. When you are exposed to sunlight or strong artificial light, it causes your brain to decrease production of melatonin and you feel more alert and brighter. Even 30-45 minutes of light exposure will affect you. Conversely, when you are in darkness your brain's melatonin levels tend to rise, making you feel sleepy. You can see why people living at high latitudes like Alaska can complain of feeling lethargic during the winter months when the dark nights are very long and the sunlit days brief—their brain melatonin levels are chronically higher and hence they feel sleepier. Exposing yourself to bright sunlight on awakening in the morning is a good way to let your brain know, "I'm supposed to be wide awake now." Keeping the lights very low in the evening before bed can help prepare your body for sleep since even modest amounts of artificial or sunlight can affect melatonin production and sleep. Unfortunately, oral melatonin supplements, though widely advertised, have not shown much promise as a sleep aid in actual research studies.

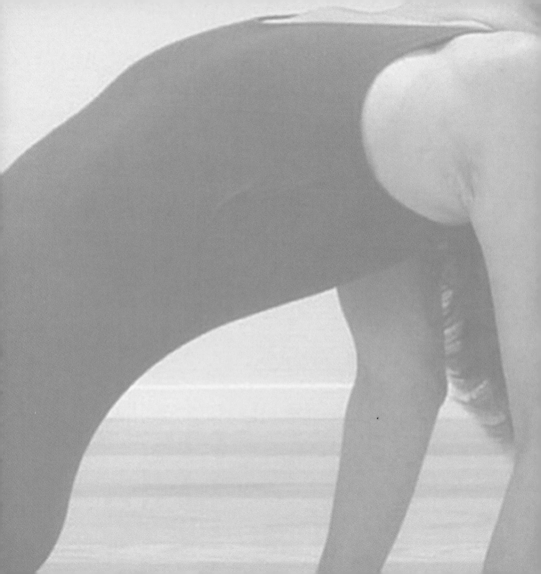

✳

Chapter Three

Insomnia: Types, Causes, and Treatments

The Types and Causes of Insomnia

Those with insomnia have abnormal sleep patterns and have difficulty falling asleep or they awaken too early and can't go back to sleep. You may have one or both problems. Most commonly, insomnia is short term, for just a few weeks, and perhaps not every night. You have chronic insomnia if your sleep problem is frequent and persists longer than a month. Those with short-term insomnia will usually have an excellent response to simple lifestyle changes, with concentration on the habits that yield good sleep. Even those with chronic insomnia can benefit from these changes.

Insomnia as a Bad Habit

Insomnia may become habitual after only a few days of poor sleep caused by stress at work, unavoidable sleep schedule changes, or a severe case of jet lag. This is the most common form of insomnia and is called "conditioned insomnia," or insomnia brought on by poor sleep habits. You've "learned" the new habit of abnormal sleep and then it becomes hard to return to your normal sleep patterns. If you suffer from this type of insomnia, you may find you are becoming increasingly anxious about sleep around bedtime and this only makes the insomnia worse. It's a downward spiral.

Insomnia Caused by Various Drugs: Prescription, Non-prescription, and Recreational

Your insomnia can also be caused by a host of sleep-disturbing drugs, including prescription medications, over-the-counter drugs, and recreational drugs (like alcohol or caffeine) that a person may have been using for years. The classic example is the person who is drinking ever-increasing amounts of coffee during the day to stay awake and ever-larger doses of alcohol at bedtime to counteract the caffeine! Both caffeine and alcohol harm our ability to sleep normally. In addition to caffeine and alcohol, other recreational drugs, such as marijuana, many non-prescription (over-the-counter) drugs like nasal decongestant tablets, and many prescription drugs end up causing about 15 % of the cases of chronic insomnia.

Alcohol deserves an extra comment because it is widely used for sleep. Unfortunately, while alcohol does cause initial sleepiness, which is why it is used, it yields only shallow, non-restorative sleep that includes suppression of your normal dream sleep.

Obviously stimulants like pseudoephedrine (a nasal decongestant tablet), non-prescription diet pills, nicotine (cigarettes), caffeine from tea or coffee, and stimulating prescription drugs like the asthma inhalers, prednisone, and some anti-depressants will interfere with normal sleep. One surprising cause of insomnia, particularly in the elderly, is the over-the-counter pain relievers that contain caffeine. Typically, the patient doesn't realize that his bedtime pain pill is what is keeping him awake!

Marijuana has a variable effect on sleep—relaxing in some, stimulating in others—but has overall negative effects for nearly everyone by reducing dream sleep; it should be avoided near bedtime. Recent studies on marijuana have also shown long-term mental function impairment, increased problems with depression, and decreased male hormone levels. We do not recommend its use unless medically supervised.

Obviously, stopping any of these sleep-disrupting agents will help with insomnia. Be sure to let your doctor know if you have a sleep problem being caused by a new medication. Insomnia may be a possible side effect to a new medication, and sometimes a simple dosage or timing adjustment, or a medication change might help.

Insomnia as a Body Clock Problem

Another common cause of insomnia is the "body clock," or circadian rhythm disorders, such as jet lag. The insomnia caused by jet lag and work shift changes is sometime referred to as "desynchronicity," illustrating that your body clock is out of synchronization with the surrounding time. Those who are trying to adapt to a new work shift schedule or a new time zone often have insomnia while their body clock adjusts. Typically, a full adjustment of your circadian body clock to a new time zone or work shift takes about ten days.

Insomnia Can Be a Sign of an Underlying Problem

Fortunately, most cases of insomnia are caused by one of the three common problems we've just outlined: learned bad sleep habits, drugs that interfere with sleep, and body clock "confusion" as in jet lag. A minority of people, however, have some underlying psychological or physical problem that is causing their insomnia or making it worse. The most common underlying problems tend to be depression or anxiety; these occur about twice as often in those complaining of insomnia.

Insomnia, Anxiety, and Depression

While most people with insomnia do not have a psychological problem, insomnia is extremely common in those with depression and anxiety disorders, and many find it their most annoying symptom. "If I could just sleep, I'd be fine. I'm really not that depressed," may be what the physician first hears. Depression and anxiety disorders frequently include insomnia as a symptom. Even when depression or anxiety disorders are adequately treated, the sleep disturbance may be the last thing to return to normal. In fact, all the patient's other symptoms may improve with just a few weeks of treatment for depression or anxiety, but the insomnia may persist for months, even though the patient is no longer depressed or anxious. If you have insomnia which does not respond to the measures suggested in this book, your physician should at least screen you for depression or anxiety, using some simple questions that look for those problems. It is also worth noting that those with sleep problems can develop depression or anxiety primarily because of their insomnia—their sleep disturbance can actually cause their depression or anxiety!

Physical Problems That Cause Insomnia

Unrefreshing sleep is a common complaint from people with significant physical health problems. Besides psychological causes like depression, insomnia may have a physical cause like untreated chronic pain, esophageal reflux, asthma, heart problems, diabetes, or sleep apnea. Those with nervous system problems like multiple sclerosis, Parkinson's disease, and dementias like Alzheimer's disease can have significant sleep disturbances. Menopausal women with hot flashes that awaken them and men with enlarged prostates who awaken to urinate frequently at night can develop severe insomnia from those annoying sleep interruptions. Both chronic fatigue syndrome and fibromyalgia patients frequently have problems with insomnia.

You can readily see that it's important to assess any obvious physical causes of insomnia, like chronic pain, early on. Treating the underlying problem along with the insomnia itself yields more successful results.

Sleep apnea literally means, "not breathing during sleep." It's more common than most suspect, affecting about 4% of people, making it about as common as diabetes. Loud snoring, fitful sleep, and even episodes of not breathing may be noted by a person's bedmate. Typically sleep apnea occurs because the person's airway intermittently collapses and actually closes off while they sleep. When they stop breathing, their brains and bodies are starved of oxygen, a condition that can cause a host of health problems over time.

Obese people, especially those with short necks, and females with very long thin necks are at higher risk of their airways closing off during sleep and causing these apnea episodes. Those with sleep apnea will often have daytime sleepiness and high blood pressure as symptoms that can provide a clue. This syndrome affects more men than women, and while obesity is a risk factor, about one-third of those with sleep apnea are not obese. Very importantly, most obese people do not have sleep apnea. The actual diagnosis of sleep apnea is made in a medical sleep test center where blood oxygen can be monitored while the patient sleeps. Sometimes weight loss can take care of the problem. If not, treatment typically involves use of a pressure mask to prevent the person's airway from closing off during the night.

Restless Leg Syndrome is surprisingly common and may affect up to 10% of the population, with men and women affected about equally. Fortunately, only a fraction of those who have this disorder find it significant. Those with this syndrome find their legs become uncomfortable or restless, primarily when they try to relax or sleep. Many sufferers also complain of odd physical sensations in their legs that are relieved by moving them, applying hot packs, squeezing the legs, or taking hot showers. They may say, "I just need to move my legs a lot to get comfortable when I go to sleep." Unfortunately, their symptoms are the worst when they attempt to relax or sleep! Their leg movements can prevent them from falling asleep and can also wake them up at night. Some may actually need to get up and walk around to feel better. Their legs may even become symptomatic sitting through a movie or on a long plane or car trip. These symptoms are often worse during pregnancy or when a person takes antidepressants. Surprisingly, iron deficiency is one common, treatable cause. There are medications that can assist in the treatment of those with severe cases of Restless Leg Syndrome.

Treatments for Insomnia

Treating insomnia is a dilemma for many physicians since their insomnia patients want help right away and often specifically request a medication that they've just seen advertised. Some physicians are unaware of the effectiveness of the lifestyle and relaxation-based treatments for insomnia that we will present in this book. But even physicians who know that lifestyle changes, better sleep habits, relaxation exercises, stretching, and affirmations are an excellent way to treat insomnia don't always make these recommendations. They may feel they don't have time or the proper materials on hand to teach everything needed. They may simply be lacking a concise presentation like this book on Ananda Yoga Therapy for insomnia to give their patients. They are tempted simply to reach for a prescription pad and give medications as a first response, without educating their patients. This is complicated by the fact that many patients will wait until their insomnia is so bad that lifestyle modification alone isn't completely effective.

Lifestyle, Attitudes, Relaxation Techniques

As we've already mentioned, positive changes in sleep-related habits and training in realistic expectations and attitudes about sleep have been shown to be as effective as medication for treating most insomnia cases. Adding a relaxation technique that is pleasant and easy to perform is also very helpful. We'll be covering these topics in great detail in the chapters that follow, and we'll discuss insomnia medications and other insomnia treatments, such as herbs, now.

Prescription Medications

Ideally these prescription medications are for short-term (a few weeks) or occasional treatment and can be used in conjunction with all the helpful advice and techniques offered in this book. Unfortunately, people's bodies may become rapidly accustomed to these medications so that over time they don't work as well. Many prescription drugs alter normal sleep patterns and can cause sleep that's less refreshing. It's possible to have withdrawal symptoms if they are stopped abruptly. The best drugs for short-term use, Ambien and Sonata, are ones that give the most normal sleep with the fewest risks and side effects. Sadly, they are also the most expensive sleep drugs, and they are often requested simply because they are widely advertised. Zolpidem (Ambien) and zaleplon (Sonata) may be too costly for those without insurance to use routinely. The benzodi-azepenes such as diazepam (Valium), alprazolam (Xanax), and temazepam (Restoril) are often employed for short-term use and are relatively inexpensive as gener-ics but have higher side-effect risks, including risks for dependency and anxiety if discontinued abruptly.

The anti-depressant trazadone (Deseryl) or mirtazapine (Remeron), which are both moderately sedating, can be given chronically and safely and in doses much lower than those used in depression treatment. The generic form of trazadone is inexpensive.

Herbs and Supplements

Melatonin, though once promising as a sleep aid, remains controver-sial. Good evidence to support its use is still lacking, and so it's not recommended for typical insom-nia treatment. However, it may have a place in the treatment of jet lag for those who are taking very long trips and have crossed at least five time zones. Some studies have found that travelers taking 5mg of melatonin at bedtime after arrival at their destination will hasten the resolution of jet lag symptoms. We suggest that you only take melatonin for jet lag at the recom-mendation of your own physician.

The amino acid tryptophan can help induce sleep, but it is not recommended in tablet form because of some fatal problems that arose with one preparation of it. However, both bananas and milk are high in tryptophan and can be eaten near bedtime. Valerian root may improve sleep but, as with many herbal products, dosing and purity remain a question. Alluna is a high quality tablet which contains valerian root.

Non-Prescription Sleep Medications

These are not recommended. Most of the liquid over-the-counter sleep drugs use alcohol as a main ingredient and, as we mentioned earlier, will cause sleepiness followed by disrupted sleep. To be blunt, don't use any products for sleep that contain alcohol. Other sleeping pills contain antihistamines, typically diphenhydramine, which is sedating but, again, does not result in normal sleep patterns. It's actually been shown that elderly patients taking over-the-counter sleeping pills have a significantly higher death rate than those taking prescription sleeping pills or nothing. If you choose to use any of these non-prescription medications, use them only occasionally or for brief periods.

When Should You See a Physician about Insomnia?

Those with chronic insomnia who don't respond to the activities in this book should consider being evaluated by a physician. We recommend this because a small number of people actually have more significant problems with their sleep, such as sleep apnea or other physical or psychological problems that should be addressed separately. In difficult cases, particularly if the patient is bothered by daytime sleepiness or if there is significant disruption of relationships, work, or enjoyable hobbies because of insomnia, evaluation by a sleep specialist may be needed.

Do You Want to Begin Sleeping Normally?

Now that you have a better understanding of sleep, and of what causes insomnia and how it's typically treated, we'll look at Ananda Yoga therapy. You'll see why it will be effective for you. The use of yoga postures as relaxation techniques, affirmations as we use in the Ananda Yoga system, and proper sleep-related habits will prove a tremendous aid. You may eliminate the need for any medication. First, let's look at how Ananda Yoga uses yoga postures, relaxation, and affirmations to help in your process of retraining and relaxing yourself for normal sleep. In Chapter Nine, we'll review all the other lifestyle changes that can help you sleep soundly and that should be used in concert with the Ananda Yoga therapy exercises.

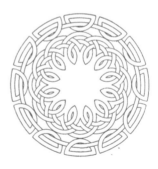

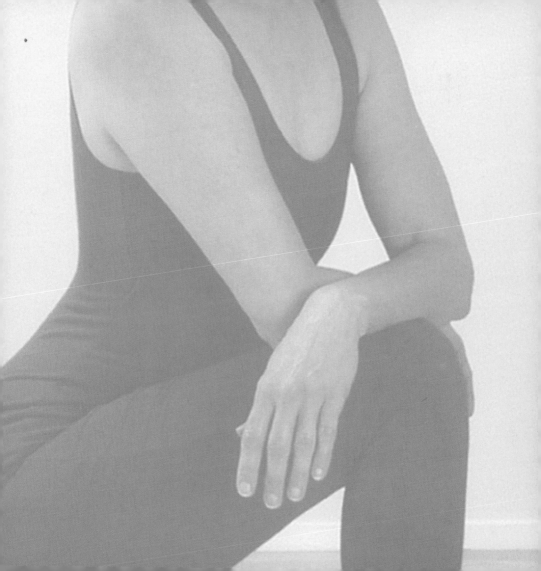

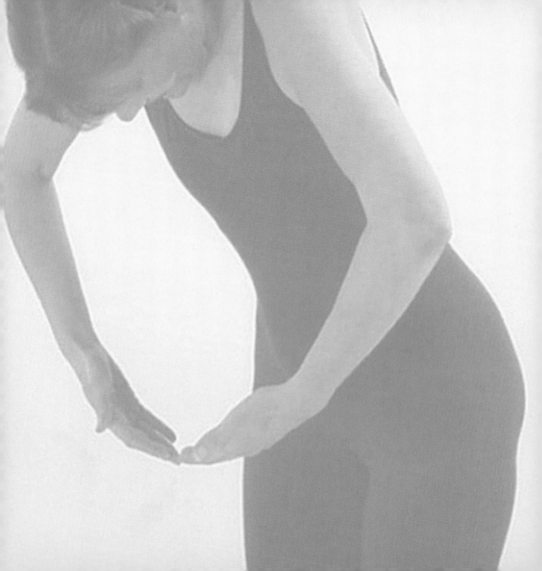

✸

Chapter Four

Ananda Yoga: An Ideal Treatment for Insomnia

What you've probably gathered from our discussion of insomnia is that the vast majority of those suffering from insomnia primarily need nothing more than retraining of their sleep habits and an effective relaxation technique to ensure they fall asleep easily. Even for those with more severe and disabling insomnia, such training can definitely help them sleep better although it may not completely solve their insomnia problem.

During the sleep-retraining phase of insomnia treatment, prescription sleeping pills are sometimes given to help the patient relax at bedtime and establish new sleep routines. However, drugs are not the only way to get a patient to relax in preparation for sleep. In our program we are using Ananda Yoga, done just before bedtime, as a sleep aid. Once you've learned our program you can do it safely for the rest of your life or just re-introduce it if your insomnia ever returns. When done in conjunction with the other habits we recommend for a great night's sleep, you will have a winning combination for overcoming insomnia.

Ananda Yoga is safe, easy, fun-to-do, and as you'll see has benefits beyond just relaxing you for sleep. Interestingly, even insurance companies have begun to explore yoga therapy and similar techniques as preventive treatments for a host of chronic medical ailments including cardiac disease. Currently there is a study underway looking at yoga postures alone as a tool for treating insomnia, and the preliminary results are promising. As you'll see,

however, Ananda Yoga is a comprehensive system for physical and mental relaxation that has several important components in addition to the actual physical yoga postures.

The unique aspect of Ananda Yoga is that it works in three different ways to get you ready for sleep. The postures involve stretching, and because they are done meditatively, they promote deep relaxation. Each yoga posture is done with an affirmation to help you draw more from the pose. This autosuggestion brings demonstrable added benefits. The breathing exercises done as part of Ananda Yoga also help deepen the level of relaxation. The three key ingredients of Ananda

Yoga: gentle stretching, affirmations, and breathing exercises have been well researched and shown to be helpful in insomnia treatment.

Relaxation and Stress Management

Insomnia is made worse by stress and emotional upset. Learning to relax consciously, as we are doing with these yoga postures, is an excellent means of stress management. Meditative relaxation has been shown beneficial in treating insomnia.

For over thirty years it's been shown repeatedly that the body has an actual relaxation response to a meditative practice like Ananda Yoga. When we are tense,

our nervous system is ready for "fight or flight." Meditative yoga postures quiet that part of the nervous system and switch on the "rest and repose" portion of the nervous system. With this quiet and inward style of yoga, a fall in blood pressure occurs, along with a decrease in heart rate and respiration rate. Even blood levels of stress hormones begin to fall.

As the nervous system relaxes, the muscles and mind relax as well. The breathing exercises included help deepen the relaxation effect and prepare both body and mind for the sleep state. Simply learning to relax "at will" can be the most important way to ensure you fall asleep quickly and easily. The more you practice a deep relaxation system like this, the faster and more deeply you'll relax. Remember we mentioned that many with insomnia have a "learned" habit of poor sleep? You're going to "learn" the habit of *conscious* physical and mental relaxation.

Affirmation

It's been shown that affirmation or autosuggestion is effective in treating many different illnesses. Autogenic training, which is very well known and studied, is one type of therapy that takes advantage of the positive effects of affirmation. Before 1950, when many fewer medication treatments for illness existed, affirmation or autosuggestion was used more widely, but interest in this technique lagged as hundreds of new and effective drugs were developed. In the last twenty years, however, we've seen a resurgence of interest in affirmations or autosuggestion as an effective and safe tool for promoting good health, particularly for disease processes where medication doesn't work well. Affirmation, done as part of Ananda Yoga, is beneficial for preparing and retraining your mind and body for refreshing sleep.

Stretching

These yoga postures are excellent, safe stretches that will get you physically relaxed and free of muscular tension. Many people are physically tight after a busy day and their bodies are "armored" into tense positions that make relaxation for sleep difficult. The Ananda Yoga system offers a balanced set of stretches that are safe, beneficial, and *pleasant* enough to do that a regular practice is easy to keep up. These yoga posture stretches may even help those with mild Restless Leg Syndrome to calm their legs.

Now let's move on to the actual practice of Ananda Yoga and you'll see the "yoga theory" behind these exercises. You'll learn the key yoga concepts that can be part of your insomnia therapy.

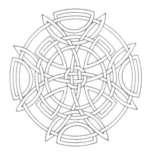

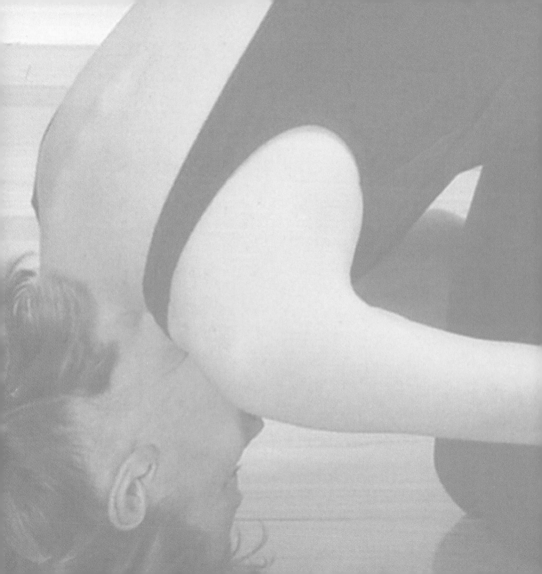

✳

Chapter Five

Keys to a Yoga Practice for Overcoming Insomnia

We've reviewed insomnia and its treatment from the standard medical perspective. Now let's look at insomnia from the perspective of traditional yoga, the broad and ancient science of which the physical yoga postures form but a small part. Yoga views health in terms of the workings of subtle energy and thought rather than just body physiology and chemistry. It's important to understand how these subtler, non-physical aspects of your being are related.

For centuries, science has viewed matter as being composed of small particles called atoms. However, within the last hundred years, scientists have found that these solid-appearing atoms are not solid after all; they are composed of energy. Therefore, energy, not solid matter, is the real building block of our universe.

Trees, rocks, water, our bodies, even the air itself—all are simply different "holding patterns" of energy.

For thousands of years traditional yoga has said much more: all energy, and hence all matter, is composed of and sustained by an even subtler form of energy, an *intelligent* energy. In Sanskrit, this subtle energy, or "life-force," is called *prana*. (Sanskrit is the language of ancient India, where yoga was developed thousands of years ago.) From the yogic perspective, in addition to being the building block for our physical bodies, prana (prah'-nah) governs all bodily functions, maintains wellness, and promotes healing. It even affects—and is affected by—our thinking. This subtle energy is the key to the body/mind connection so often discussed today. Although it is not yet recognized by Western medical science, many traditional healing methods, including acupuncture, are designed to influence this energy directly to promote health and wellness.

Yoga says that health problems result when the flow of energy is blocked or out of harmony.[1] Yoga would say that insomnia, for example, results from energy that is agitated, out of control, or

---

1 From this point onward, we will use the more familiar word "energy" (or sometimes "sublte energy") to refer to prana. Since we are not also using "energy" in the more familiar sense of "calories" in this book, there should be no confusion.

perhaps locked into disharmonious patterns. Although a person might not perceive out-of-control energy, he or she would experience associated symptoms such as physical restlessness, preoccupation with negative or bothersome thoughts, poor concentration, and emotional agitation.

Yoga offers many techniques that help harness subtle energy and restore its harmonious flow; the physical yoga positions (asanas) are the most visible of these. Asana (aah'-sah-nah) actually means "physical posture" in Sanskrit. Through stretching and relaxation, the asanas offer many important physical benefits; however, the postures' greatest value lies in their ability to promote and harmonize the smooth, free flow of energy in the body.

In fact, any bodily position affects the flow of energy. You can easily experience this yourself: sit up straight, take several deep breaths, smile, and lift your gaze slightly upward. Notice how you feel. Now slouch into your chair, round your spine, frown, and look downward. It's the same body as a moment ago, but you feel different—physically and mentally. Why? In yoga, we would say it is caused primarily by a change in the energy. The first position encouraged a free, upward flow of energy—which yoga says is connected with feelings of happiness—whereas the second inhibited it, and even promoted a downward flow.

Similarly, each asana has a specific effect on your energy, and through it, your state of mind and health. For example, both the asanas shown here help release energy trapped in the legs, which is a common contributor to restlessness, and hence to insomnia. Of course, yoga postures are not magic pills; however, their effects can be quite deep once you learn to use not only your body, but the power of your mind, as we'll explain below. In this way, asanas

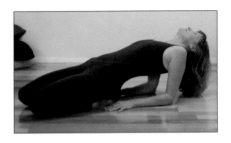

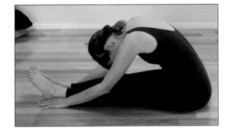

and other yoga techniques can be highly effective tools for harmonizing your energy, with the result that you will feel calmer, more positive, and healthier.

Learning to control your subtle energy and thoughts is the heart of Ananda Yoga practice, which forms the basis for our therapeutic approach. Working deeply with energy requires considerable training and experience; the simple approach we offer here will help you build a foundation for this deeper work (*see Chapter Eleven: Next Steps with Ananda Yoga*).

General Principles for Practicing Ananda Yoga

In Ananda Yoga practice, you consciously involve all three levels of your being: physical, mental/feeling, and spiritual.

The physical level of the practice, means always moving your body gracefully, with sensitive awareness of what you're doing. When doing the asanas, strive for comfort and relaxation—even in more challenging asanas—rather than outward achievement or picture-book form. This is not a sports competition! Yes, you want to go deep into the stretches, but always honor your limitations and never strain. Strain causes tension or even injury, not harmony—and certainly will not help you sleep.

Involving the mental/feeling level of your being means not only concentrating fully on what you're doing with your body, but immersing your mind in the attitudes promoted by the postures. Try to feel those attitudes. To help you in this, Ananda Yoga offers an affirmation for each asana, specially designed to reinforce the particular mental and energetic effects that the asana promotes. *(See "Keys to Practicing Affirmations.")*

The spiritual level is especially important. Whatever you wish to call it—soul, Self, our highest potential, light, divine essence, God—each of us knows intuitively that we have a higher reality than the body and personality. The entire science of yoga is designed to bring you into alignment with your own higher reality, for that is the key to harmony and well-being on all levels. Therefore, do the postures with a feeling of ever-increasing harmony with that higher reality. This is the subtlest aspect of the practice, but it is not mysterious. It is you! Increasing your attunement with it will do more to harmonize the flow of subtle energy than anything else you can do.

Re-establishing wellness is often a gradual process. Experience with yoga over millennia has shown, however, that those who persevere and follow common-sense safety guidelines *(see Practical Guidelines for Your Therapeutic Practice)* can expect to find greater harmony and wellness on many levels of their being.

Modern research has documented that affirmations can play a powerful role in wellness. They can be particularly effective for insomnia, because it often involves such a strong mental/emotional/psychological component.

Affirmations are statements of higher truths that help re-educate and "reprogram" the subconscious mind by changing harmful habits of thought into helpful habits. More importantly, they help us attune our minds with natural states of relaxation, health, harmony, and vitality—and above all, with our divine essence.

In Ananda Yoga, each asana is paired with a specific affirmation designed to enhance the benefits of the asana. The asana in turn strengthens your experience of the affirmation. For maximum effectiveness, the asana should be done without strain, and the affirmation should be used with both concentration and feeling as you hold the physical position. Let's look at these two elements: concentration and feeling.

Concentration is vital to success in anything. Just as the focused beam of a laser is more powerful than the dispersed rays of an ordinary light bulb, a focused mind will charge your words with power. If your mind is restless or scattered, repeat the affirmation aloud to gain focus. Once your mind is focused, repeat the affirmation silently—over and over, with increasing concentration—to direct your efforts inwardly to the core of your being. With silent affirmation, do not move the tongue or lips.

Feeling, too, is vital for affirmation. It is a calm, inward sense of clarity or upliftment, such as when you are inspired by nature, by another person, or by a great work of art. It is different from emotion, which tends to carry you outward into agitation or excitement. Bringing feeling into an affirmation is far superior to mere mechanical repetition; it is the key to receiving the best results from your practice. Let's look at some examples of this.

Remember our earlier example of sitting up straight, breathing deeply, smiling, and lifting your gaze to help boost your mood? These four gestures will be even more effective if you also consciously strive to *feel* happier and affirm with calm certainty, "I feel great!"

Similarly, to get the most out of an asana, try to *experience* the quality suggested by its affirmation.

For example, when affirming peacefulness, strive to *feel* your inner peace increasing as you repeat the affirmation. When affirming that you're in command of your own energies, *be* strongly and confidently in charge; bring your calm determination to the fore. Although this use of "feeling" is a subtle aspect of Ananda Yoga practice, it is very important for bringing about the results you seek.

If you are new to the practice of affirmation, it may take practice to get beyond the thought that affirmations are "just pretending." Remember, however, that affirmation is not a mere "sales job," an attempt to convince yourself of something. Rather, it's about replacing old, unhelpful attitudes with new, positive ones that reflect a higher octave of who you are. You need not create that higher octave. It's *already* a truth of your own being; you just need to begin to experience it as your moment-to-moment reality. This takes concentration, feeling, and whole-hearted participation. Once you realize that your state of mind is within your control, your affirmations will gain tremendous power—and you will feel tremendously empowered in your own life.

Practical Guidelines for Your
Therapeutic Practice

1. Practice on an empty stomach: wait at least 3 hours after a large meal, and ideally 1-2 hours after a snack. (In this book, you will be practicing just before bedtime. If you have had a late dinner, or if a small snack is part of your bedtime routine, simply practice gently and sensitively as common sense dictates, especially with any postures that put pressure on the abdomen.)

2. Practice in a warm, quiet, well-ventilated place without bright light of any kind.

3. Wear loose, comfortable clothing. For this insomnia routine, your pajamas may be just fine.

4. Never strain. If a posture is uncomfortable for you, modify it to suit your body rather than trying to force your body into some "ideal" position. (For many of the postures, easier modifications are given.) Never ignore tensions that keep you from stretching farther; indeed, concentrate on them and try to relax them away. Use props (cushions, blankets, etc.) as needed to accomplish this.

5. Honor any cautions given for the poses. Keep in mind that we offer only some very general cautions; for space reasons, we could

not include a comprehensive list of restrictions. Use common sense, and when in doubt, consult your physician.

6. Keep your breath flowing smoothly and naturally in all poses. Holding your breath or breathing unevenly while in a posture is a sign of strain, which draws you away from relaxation, harmony, and sleep.

7. Practice these exercises meditatively, with a sense of patient, relaxed, alert, inward awareness. Do not worry about whether the exercises will end your insomnia, for that very thought will dilute the effects of the exercises. Simply practice them with a sense of complete involvement in—and enjoyment of—what you are doing.

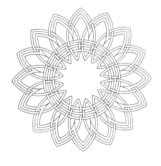

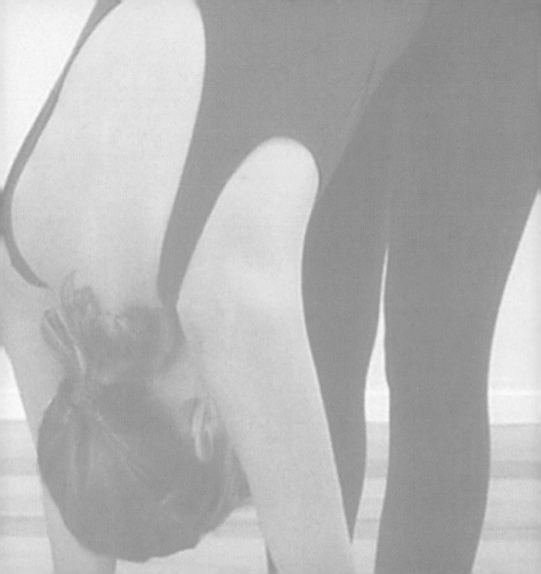

✻

Chapter Six

Exercises for Preventing and Relieving Insomnia

We offer two brief Ananda Yoga routines designed to help you prepare for sleep by eliminating restlessness and relaxing your body and mind:

- *Main Routine*—Once you learn it, this takes about fifteen minutes. Then you get into bed for the final exercise, which is designed to take you directly into sleep.

- *Short Routine*—Once you learn it, this takes about five minutes.

Then you get into bed for the final exercise, which is designed to take you directly into sleep.

Below are summaries of these two routines and how to use them; detailed instructions for all the exercises are given in Chapter Seven. You can find additional information on Ananda Yoga Therapy for insomnia at www.AnandaYoga.org.

How to Use the Routines

Begin with the Main Routine, practicing it each night immediately before going to bed. Once your difficulties with insomnia diminish—which might happen right away—switch to the Short Routine. In time, you may find that just 1:2 Breathing (the last exercise listed in both routines) or one of the additional "into sleep" techniques described below after step twelve is enough to take you into relaxing sleep. Anytime that you feel particularly agitated or "wound up" at bedtime, use the Main Routine.

Shown below each pose title are suggested lengths of time to spend with each exercise. Feel free to increase those times according to what you find to be beneficial.

Before beginning your practice, make all preparations for sleep—brush your teeth, set your alarm clock, whatever you ordinarily do—so the last exercise can take you into sleep. Ideally, do not wear glasses or contact lenses during your practice.

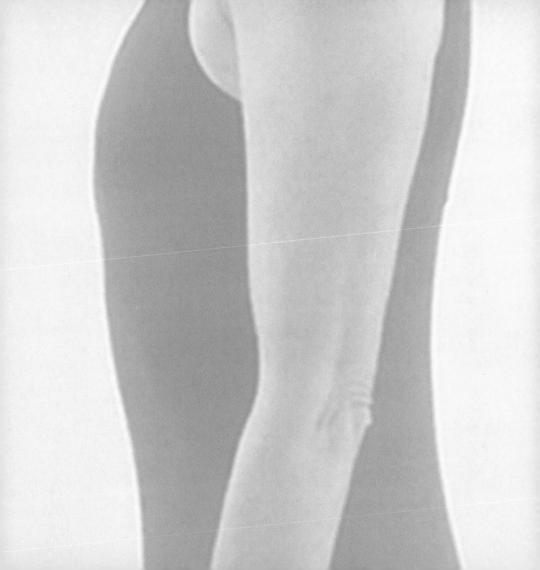

Main Routine

1. 20-Part Body Recharging—
see page 90

2. Full Yogic Breath in Mountain Pose (3-6 breaths)—*see page 94*

3. Full Yogic Breath Flow (5 breaths)—*see page 96*

a. Mountain Pose, exhale to forward bend

b. Use palms to lift energy up through body

c. Complete inhalation with stretch

d. Exhale and wipe away tension

4. Lunge
(30 seconds each side)—*see page 100*

5. Hare Pose
(at least 30 seconds)—*see page 104*

Affirmation: "I am master of my energy, I am master of myself."

6. Child Pose
(30 seconds)—*see page 108*

Affirmation: "I relax from outer involvement into my inner haven of peace."

7. Supine Firm Pose
(at least 30 seconds)—*see page 112*

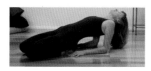

Affirmation: "Energetic movement, or unmoving peace: The choice is mine alone. The choice is mine."

8. Posterior Stretching Pose
(30 seconds to 2 minutes)—*see page 118*

Affirmation: "I am safe, I am sound. All good things come to me; they give me peace."

9. Fish Pose
(30 seconds)—*see page 122*

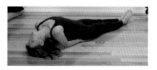

Affirmation: "My soul floats on waves of cosmic light."

10. Supine Twist
(at least 30 seconds each side)—*see page 124*

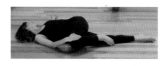

Affirmation: "I open to the flow of God's life within me."

11. Optional: The Calming Breath
(as long as desired)—*see page 128*

12. 1:2 Breathing in Corpse Pose (for as long as needed to attain sleep)—*see page 131*

Additional "into Sleep" Techniques
(select as desired)

♦20-Part Progressive Relaxation (one or more passes)—*see page 134*

♦Visualization with Breath Control (6–12 times)—*see page 136*

♦Withdrawal from Outward Awareness—*see page 137*

♦Affirmation (as desired, with or without breath control)—*see page 138*

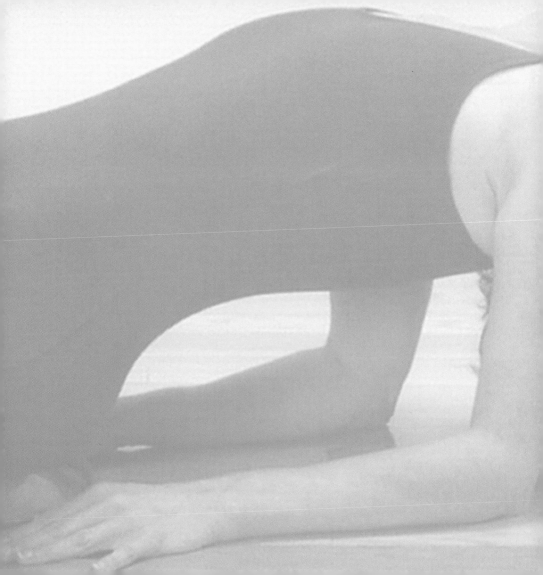

Short Routine

1. Full Yogic Breath Flow
(5 breaths)—*see page 96*

a. Mountain Pose, exhale to forward bend

b. Use palms to lift energy up through body

c. Complete inhalation with stretch

d. Exhale and wipe away tension

2. Lunge
(30 seconds each side)—*see page 100*

3. Hare Pose
(at least 30 seconds)—*see page 104*

Affirmation: "I am master of my energy, I am master of myself."

4. Child Pose
(30 seconds)—*see page 108*

Affirmation: "I relax from outer involvement into my inner haven of peace."

5. Supine Firm Pose
(at least 30 seconds)—*see page 112*

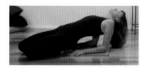

Affirmation: "Energetic movement, or unmoving peace: The choice is mine alone. The choice is mine."

6. Supine Twist
(at least 30 seconds each side)—*see page 124*

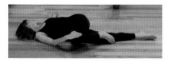

Affirmation: "I open to the flow of God's life within me."

7. 1:2 Breathing in Corpse Pose
(for as long as needed to attain sleep)—*see page 131*

Additional "into Sleep" Techniques
(select as desired)

♦20-Part Progressive Relaxation (one or more passes)—*see page 134*

♦Visualization with Breath Control (6–12 times)—*see page 136*

♦Withdrawal from Outward Awareness—*see page 137*

♦Affirmation (as desired, with or without breath control)—*see page 138*

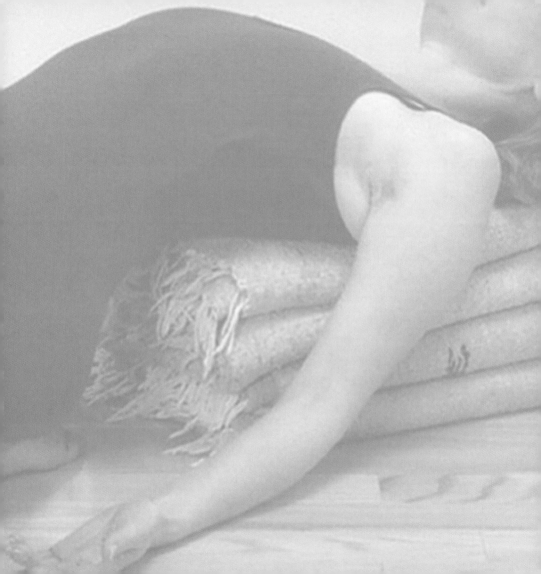

Chapter Seven

✳

Instructions for the Exercises

Once you no longer need the detailed instructions below, it will be more convenient to use the summaries of the Short Routine and Main Routine in Chapter Six.

Breathing Basics

According to the science of yoga, one common cause of poor sleep (and many other health problems) is improper breathing. The following two basic breathing techniques are used in both the Main Routine and the Short Routine; they promote relaxation and better health generally.

Diaphragmatic Breathing

Many people breathe by moving only the chest wall, taking shallow breaths that deprive them of adequate oxygen. Scientific studies have also shown that chest breathing induces stress and restlessness. It is far healthier to breathe with the diaphragm, so that the abdomen moves in and out with the breath. (The chest moves, too, but not as much as the abdomen.) This Diaphragmatic Breathing has the opposite effect: it both relaxes you and enables your lungs to absorb more oxygen.

The diaphragm leads the inhalation by moving downward, gently pushing the abdomen outward and inflating the lungs (*see top drawing*). When the diaphragm moves upward, the abdomen moves inward and air is squeezed out of the lungs, i.e., you exhale (*bottom drawing*).

Diaphragmatic Breathing is easiest to observe if you lie on your back on the floor: Place one hand over

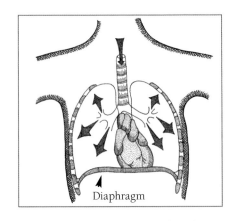

The diaphragm is a dome-shaped sheet of muscle and tendon located just beneath your lungs.

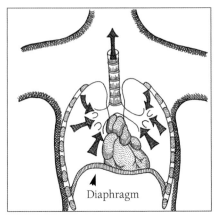

your navel, close your eyes, and relax your entire body. Breathe naturally, not controlling your breath. Notice how your abdomen lifts your hand with each inhalation and relaxes down with each exhalation. These movements are caused by the downward (toward the pelvis) and upward (toward the head) movements of the diaphragm, respectively. It's how you naturally breathe when you are relaxed. Notice that the rib cage, too, expands somewhat with each inhalation; this is natural, but unless you breathe deeply, you will feel more activity in the abdomen than in the rib cage. Notice also how little effort it takes when you breathe diaphragmatically; contrast that with breathing by expanding your chest and leaving your abdomen completely out of the process. The latter takes a lot more work!

When you are sitting or standing, much the same thing occurs (although the lower ribs expand and contract slightly more than when lying down). However, due to habitual slouching—or tensing the abdomen out of a desire to look thin—many people breathe only with the chest. It takes awareness and practice to keep the abdominal muscles relaxed, but as noted above, it's healthier and more calming to breathe that way—and it takes less physical effort, too.

Diaphragmatic Breathing reduces stress, relaxes your body and mind, better oxygenates your cells, and increases the effectiveness of the exercises below. In fact, if you breathe this way throughout your day, you will soon form new breathing habits that will provide definite health benefits for the rest of your life.

The Full Yogic Breath

A diaphragmatic inhalation (as described in Diaphragmatic Breathing section) is the first phase of the Full Yogic Breath, also known as the Three-Part Breath. As you continue to inhale after the abdomen expands, the lower ribs will expand (second phase), and finally the upper chest will expand (third phase) as you finish the inhalation. The full yogic exhalation immediately follows (do not hold the breath), also in three phases: first the upper chest relaxes to a normal position, then the lower ribs relax inward, and finally the abdomen returns to its initial position. Do not squeeze with the abdominal muscles to complete the exhalation; let them relax. The exhalations should be the same length as inhalations unless we instruct you otherwise.

Full Yogic Breaths should be comfortably deep, with no sense of strain, neither filling the lungs to maximum capacity nor squeezing them to nearly empty. Take care not to arch the spine as you inhale; you should instead feel the torso expand to all sides rather than feel the abdomen and rib cage push dramatically forward. Breathe slowly and with a sense of ease, with each inhalation and each exhalation lasting about 5 seconds (more or less according to comfort). The three phases should flow smoothly, one into the next, rather than being rigid or separated. Think of the inhalation as a gradual upward expansion of the torso, and the exhalation as a downward relaxation.

The Full Yogic Breath is an excellent way to take control of your energy and, simultaneously, to relax. In time, you might be able to dispense with the asanas and simply use the Full Yogic Breath to prepare for sleep. However, if your breathing habits have been poor (e.g., if you've been a chest breather rather than a diaphragmatic breather), it may take some practice to get comfortable with the Full Yogic Breath. While you're learning it, therefore, feel free to use Diaphragmatic Breathing as needed—both in the exercises below and throughout your day.

Guidelines for Breathing during the Exercises

Unless otherwise instructed, please:

- Begin your routine with the Full Yogic Breath and use it in the exercises as long as you are feeling agitation. Once your energy has calmed down, move into Diaphragmatic Breathing.

- Breathe through your nose, with nose and face relaxed, and without undue noise—don't "sniff" your inhalations or "snort" your exhalations.

- Breathe as slowly as you can without discomfort.

- Take smooth and relaxed breaths, with no strain or jerkiness.

- Breathe evenly—with equal-length inhalations and exhalations. (One exercise uses a variant in which the exhalations are twice as long as the inhalations; we point that out when it comes up.)

- Breathe naturally—inhale fully, but not to near bursting; do not hold the breath unnaturally after any inhalation or exhalation; and do not attempt to squeeze as much air as possible out of the lungs on exhalation.

General Asana Instructions

The exercises below are safe for most people, and basic cautions are given for certain conditions. For some exercises, you may need one or more firm blankets or cushions, a straight-backed chair, and a yoga strap (you can use a necktie, scarf, or long sock instead).

For best results—and if you have the time—hold the poses for a longer period of time than suggested below, provided there's no strain in doing so.

Some Yoga Terminology

Straight spine: A healthy spine has a gentle inward curve in the lower back, a gentle outward curve in the back of the chest, and another gentle inward curve in the neck. When the spine has these natural curves (and none of them are excessive), yogis call it a "straight spine." Note: different bodies may have different amounts of natural curvature.

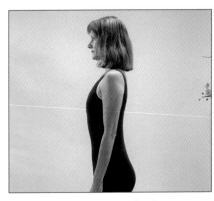

Sit-bones: These are the bony protuberances on the bottom of your pelvis, the parts that complain when you sit too long on a hard surface. Anatomists call them "ischial tuberosities"; we'll use the simpler term "sit-bones."

Tuck the pelvis: In the backward-bending asanas, you will be instructed to "tuck your pelvis," i.e., drop your tailbone as though you were tucking your tail between your legs, but without thrusting the entire pelvis forward. This will help keep your spine long and pre-vent excessive bending in the lumbar (lower back) region.

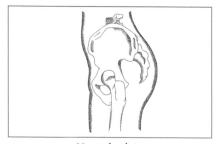

Neutral pelvis

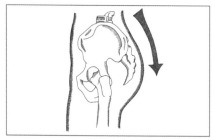

Tucked pelvis

Closed, uplifted eyes: Stand or sit upright and gaze softly at a point a few feet in front of you, slightly above the horizon. Then close your eyelids, continuing to gaze in that same direction. Do not try to see anything, however, or lift your gaze so high that you strain your eye muscles. Simply relax your eyes slightly upward as though they were drawn naturally toward that point. This "closed, uplifted eyes" position is a classical yoga technique that gently nudges your awareness toward a calm, relaxed, uplifted state of awareness. It will become more comfortable as your eye muscles grow accustomed to it. Whenever indicated in these routines, close your eyes and gently lift them into this position.

Cautions: Some physical conditions call for special care in certain poses. For these we have used the following shorthand terms: "Spinal injuries" refers to conditions such as painful bulging or ruptured discs, pinched nerves, severe back pain, etc.—as well as recurrent or chronic strain—anywhere in the spine, including the neck. "Eye, ear, or sinus problems" refers to diseases or inflammations of areas in the head, such as glaucoma, detached retina, earache, sinus congestion/infection, headache, etc. "Cardiovascular problems" refers to hardening of the arteries, heart disease, high blood pressure, history of stroke or heart attack, etc. Anyone with serious health problems of any kind should practice only under the supervision of a qualified yoga instructor and with a release from his or her physician.

The Primary Exercises

Following is the Main Routine. The Short Routine consists of the exercises marked with an "✳", done in the same order as they appear below. The Additional "into Sleep" Techniques follow.

1.   20-Part Body Recharging

Here, you will forcibly take control of your energy by tensing, then relaxing, various body parts, using concentration, visualization, and willpower. How hard should you tense? If you feel relatively relaxed to begin with, then tense with only light to medium tension, so as not to be agitating. But if you feel restless and "wired," tensing hard will help you release the restlessness.

The exercise has four phases:

Phase 1: Inhale deeply, then hold the breath and tense the entire body. Then relax as you exhale.

Phase 2: Next, tense and relax the 20 individual body parts, one part at a time in the order shown in the photo at right: Slowly tense each part; visualize energy flowing to the center of the body part to cause tension. Tense only that one body part and no others. (It takes practice to be able to isolate your muscles in this way.) Then slowly relax as you visualize energy withdrawing from the body part into the center of your body. Take 2–3 seconds to tense fully, and 2–3 seconds to relax fully.

Let the breath flow on its own, but do keep it flowing rather than holding it. Tense and relax the body parts in the order indicated in the accompanying drawing, isolating each part.

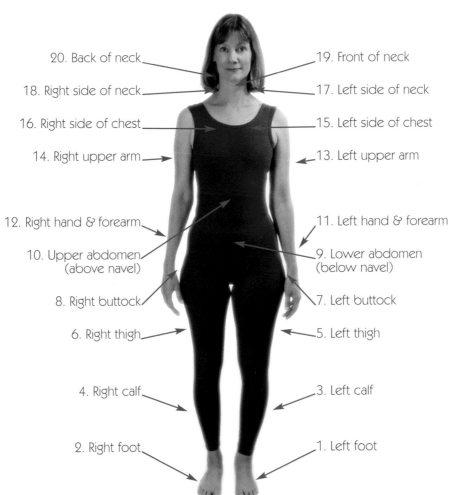

20. Back of neck

19. Front of neck

18. Right side of neck

17. Left side of neck

16. Right side of chest

15. Left side of chest

14. Right upper arm

13. Left upper arm

12. Right hand & forearm

11. Left hand & forearm

10. Upper abdomen (above navel)

9. Lower abdomen (below navel)

8. Right buttock

7. Left buttock

6. Right thigh

5. Left thigh

4. Right calf

3. Left calf

2. Right foot

1. Left foot

91

Phase 3: Next, in rapid succession, tense each of the 20 body parts, one at a time in the same order as in Phase 2. This time, do not relax any of them; rather, accumulate tension in the body as you move upward. When you reach the top, your entire body will be tensed.

Phase 4: After holding the tension briefly at the top, relax all four parts of the neck simultaneously and release your chin to your chest. Then in rapid succession, relax the other 16 body parts in reverse order: right side of the chest, left side of the chest, right upper arm, left upper arm, and so on, all the way down to the feet.

In time, you may enjoy doing Phase 3 over the course of one long inhalation, and Phase 4 over the course of the ensuing long exhalation.

It takes practice to develop the body awareness and concentration needed for this exercise. The results, however, are definitely worth the work required to learn it: you will be much more in control of your energy, as well as more relaxed. In fact, you can use it at any time of the day to clear the mind and relax tension.

Cautions

Those with cardiovascular problems should be especially careful to keep the breath flowing and begin with light tension, increasing the tension over time as they learn to practice without unduly raising blood pressure. Pregnant or menstruating women should tense the upper and lower abdomen only lightly, according to their level of comfort.

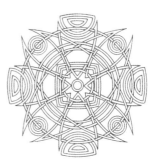

2. Full Yogic Breath in Mountain Pose

Stand upright with your feet hip-width apart. Place equal weight on both feet, and equal weight on the balls of your feet and your heels. Align your body so that a vertical line through the center of your ear intersects the centers of the shoulder, hip, knee, and ankle joints. (Ask a friend to help you find this alignment.) Keep your chin level and your spine straight. Lengthen upward through your entire body, relaxing your abdomen and the front, sides, and back of your rib cage. This is the proper posture whenever you are standing; it is called Mountain Pose (*see figure at right*).

With closed, uplifted eyes, take 3–6 slow Full Yogic Breaths, feeling a wave of expansion moving up through your torso with each inhalation, and relaxing (without slouching or losing your height) with each exhalation.

Note: Due to past postural habits, you might feel unnatural in Mountain Pose at first. Do not try to perfect this pose immediately; rather, slowly move closer to this ideal over weeks and months. Practice Mountain Pose throughout your day: while waiting in line, washing dishes, standing in conversation with others, etc. By cultivating proper posture, you will reduce or eliminate some of the tensions and muscle imbalances that

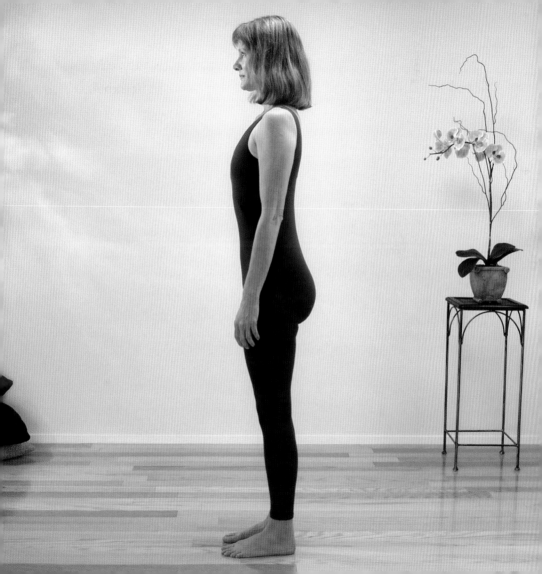

contribute to insomnia, headaches, and a host of other discomforts.

✳ 3. Full Yogic Breath Flow

This exercise relaxes muscular restriction in and around the diaphragm, ribs, and chest, helping the breath—and subtle energy—flow freely and naturally. Do it with a sense of relaxation, as though cleansing the body and mind of "tension toxins." Throughout the exercise, feel that you are harmonizing the energy flows in the body.

In Mountain Pose, take a full yogic inhalation. On the full yogic exhalation, bend your knees slightly and slowly hinge forward from the hips, ending in "rag doll position" as you finish your exhalation. If your spine is healthy, it's okay to let it round gently—through relaxation, not through straining to reach lower—as you bend forward. Try always to keep a sense of length in the spine, so it doesn't feel "scrunched" (figure a, page 98).

Upon reaching bottom, immediately begin a full yogic inhalation as you slowly straighten back up, drawing your hands up the front of the body (palms up, not quite touching the body), with elbows out to the sides. As you bring your hands up, feel that you are smoothing your breath and lifting energy up through the body (figure b, page

98). Complete your inhalation by stretching upward, coming up on the balls of your feet and opening your chest and shoulders *(figure c, page 99)*. Hold the stretch for 2–3 counts before starting to exhale down out of the stretch.

As you exhale, glide your hands down the front of the body (palms down, not quite touching the body—*figure d, page 99)*, as though soothing your body by wiping away all tension, anxiety, and restlessness—mental as well as physical—as you return to the full forward bending position.

Continue for 4 more breaths. After your last upward stretch, slowly exhale and return to Mountain Pose by gracefully sweeping your hands out to your sides in a wide arc as though surrounding yourself with an aura of peace.

Caution

If you have a spinal injury, either keep your spine straight throughout this exercise (for minor injuries) or do this exercise without bending forward at all, using the hands and the breath as described above.

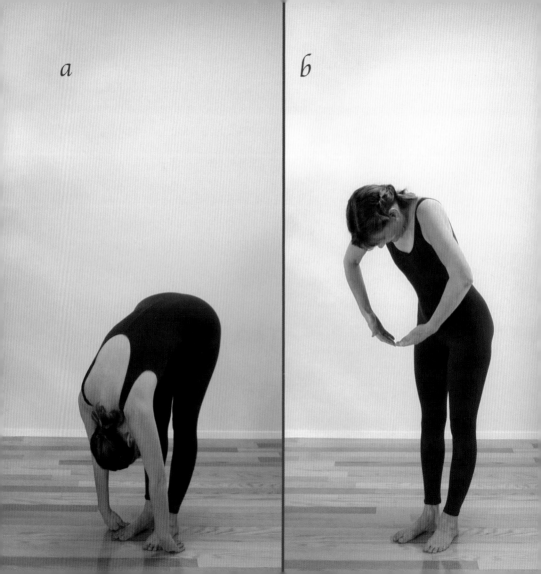

a

b

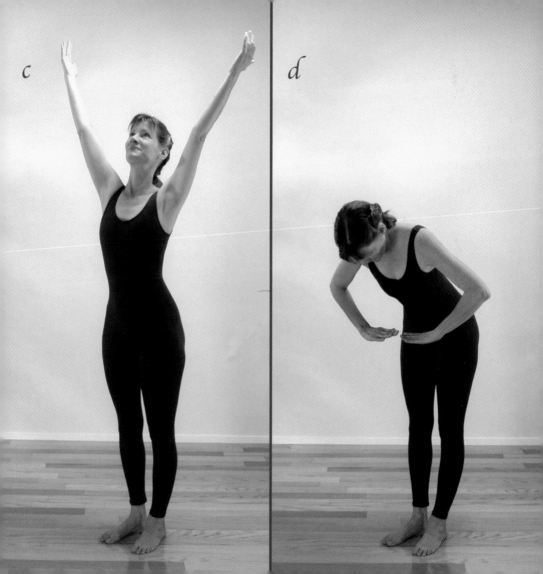

c

d

✳ 4. Lunge

Step your left foot forward, right foot back, and come down into a lunging position: left knee directly above left ankle, right knee on the floor, and right foot back far enough that you feel a definite stretch through the front of your right thigh, hip, and groin. (If this is uncomfortable for your right knee, cushion it on a folded blanket.) Keep your spine upright and straight, and your pelvis tucked to avoid overarching your lower back. Interlace your fingers on your left thigh and soften your shoulders. Spread open across your chest and shoulders, without squeezing your shoulder blades together. Concentrate on relaxing throughout the pelvic region as you release it toward the floor with each exhalation.

Hold this position for 30 seconds. Rest briefly, then repeat to the other side.

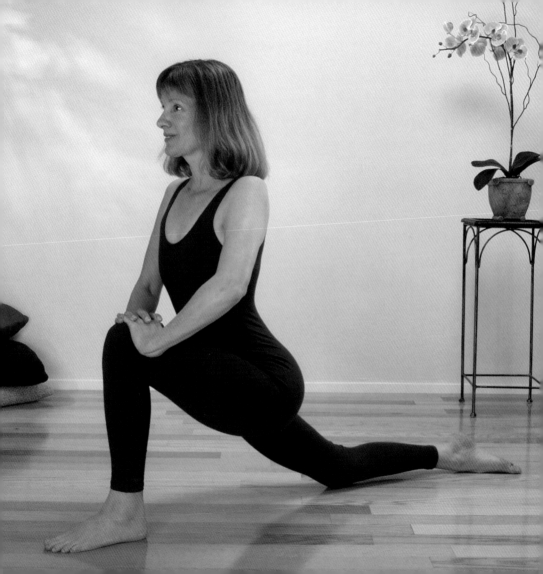

For a gentler stretch, bend forward and rest your forearms on your knee (*figure a*). Or gentler still, place your hands on the floor on either side of your left foot, staying up on your fingertips to keep your chest open and breath flowing easily (*figure b*). For either variation, keep your entire spine straight (i.e., counter any tendency to round the spine and/or arch the neck backward).

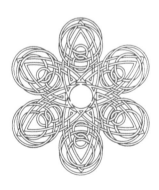

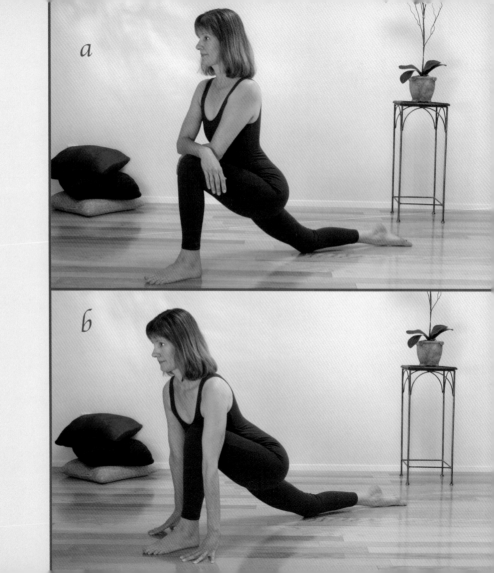

✳ **5.** Hare Pose

Sit on your heels, thighs parallel and arms at your sides. Inhale as you lengthen your spine, then exhale as you bend forward from the hips, leading with your chest. Keep your spine long as you lay your abdomen over your thighs and rest your forehead on the floor and arms by your sides, palms up. Relax briefly in this initial position (*Child Pose; see figure a*).

Now grasp your heels, with your fingertips on the inner heels and insteps, and thumbs on the outside edges of your feet (*figure b*). Bring your forehead as close to your knees as is comfortable, and place the crown of your head on the floor. Continue holding your heels as you inhale and lift your buttocks, stretching your arms straight. Rest only a small amount of weight on the crown of your head; most of your weight should be on your legs (*figure c*).

Continue lifting through the legs and feel the stretch in your arms, shoulders, and back. This pose helps you gain control over the energy in the entire body—especially the spine, which is the central channel for the flow of subtle energy. With closed, uplifted eyes, hold the pose for at least 30 seconds, affirming,

*"I am master of my energy,
I am master of myself."*

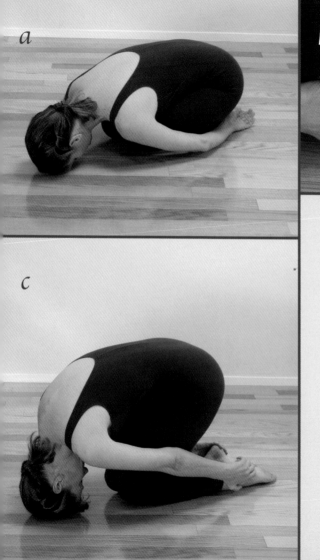

a

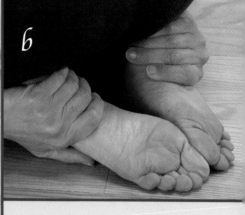

b

c

I am master
of my energy,
I am master
of myself.

To exit the pose, slowly lower your buttocks back down to your heels, release your hands, and relax completely in Child Pose.

Variations

If you cannot grasp your heels, loop a yoga strap around your heels and hold the strap with your hands, effectively lengthening your arms (*figure a*). Or, hold one wrist with the other hand behind your thighs, and stretch forward against the resistance of the backs of your thighs.

If your neck is vulnerable to injury or your knees are uncomfortable in the pose, you can use a chair: rest your torso on your thighs, grasp the chair's rear legs, then stretch forward to create a "dynamic resistance" effect similar to that of the standard Hare Pose (*figure b*).

Cautions

Avoid turning your head to either side while in this pose. Avoid this pose if you have recent spinal injuries, or eye, ear, or sinus problems.

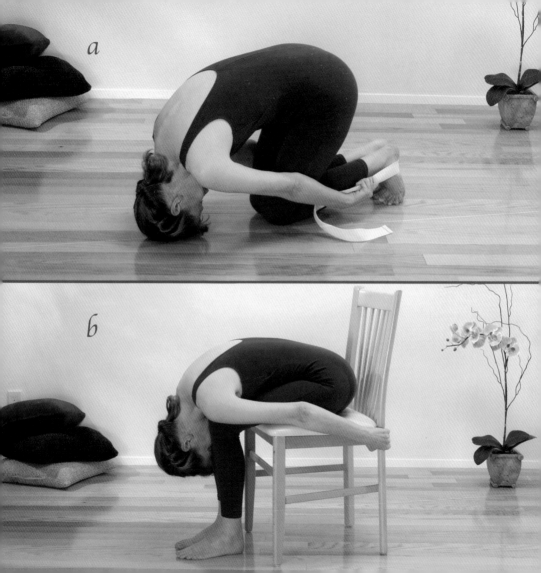

a

b

✳ 6. Child Pose

Remain in Child Pose and relax your entire body, especially your arms, shoulders, upper back, and legs. Let the weight of your torso squeeze all tensions out of your legs.

Close and uplift your eyes, and feel your breath massaging and relaxing your back and shoulders. Remain in this pose for 30 seconds, affirming,

"I relax from outer involvement into my inner haven of peace."

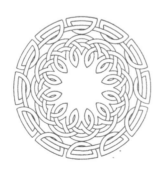

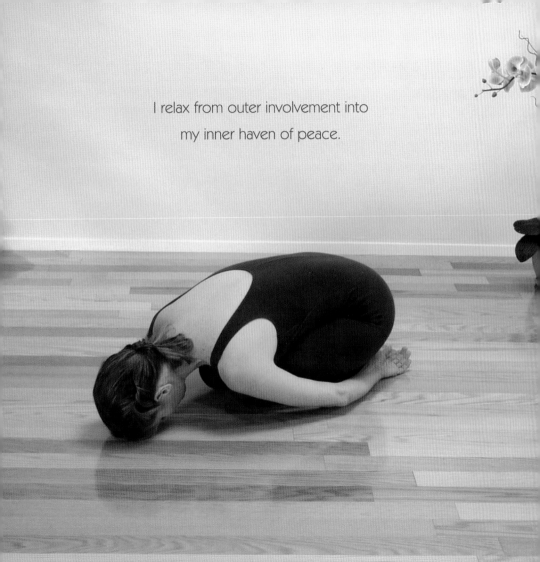

I relax from outer involvement into

my inner haven of peace.

Variations

If your knees are uncomfortable when flexed like this, you can decrease the flexion by placing a cushion between your ankles and buttocks (*figure a*). If your ankles are uncomfortable, you can lessen the stretch by placing a rolled towel under the fronts of your ankles (*also figure a*). If you like, bring your arms up beside your head and rest your head on your forearms.

Pregnant women and overweight persons should move their knees apart in this pose for greater comfort.

If none of the preceding variations is comfortable for you, sit on a chair and bend forward, resting your torso on your thighs. Relax your neck completely and let your arms hang loosely to the floor. If needed, place a cushion under your chest so you can deeply relax (*figure b*).

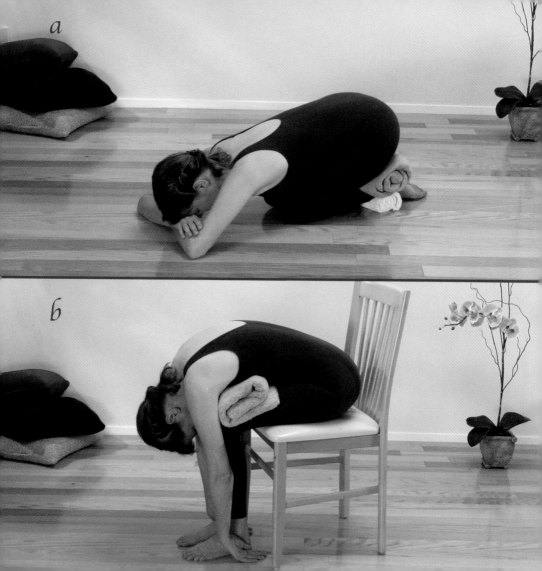

a

b

* 7. Supine Firm Pose

Those who can be comfortable and relaxed in this pose will find it very effective for relief of restlessness. Since not everyone finds comfort and relaxation in the basic pose that we're about to describe, we will also offer a variety of easier variations.

Sit on your heels with thighs parallel. Lean back and place your palms on the floor 12-18 inches behind your toes, shoulder-width apart with fingers pointing toward your feet. Tuck your pelvis and slowly lower yourself onto your elbows. At all times, keep your pelvis tucked and your knees together and on the floor. If you cannot come all the way down onto your elbows, simply come down as far as is comfortable. Align your neck with the rest of your spine.

Relax and "open" the entire front of your body—especially the thighs and hip region, where get-up-and-go energy often causes the legs to tense at the mere thought of moving. With continual stress, such tension becomes chronic and disturbs sleep. Don't let such unconscious reactions rule you. Close and uplift your eyes, and hold this pose for at least 30 seconds—up to 2-3 minutes if comfortable—consciously releasing tension in the legs and affirming,

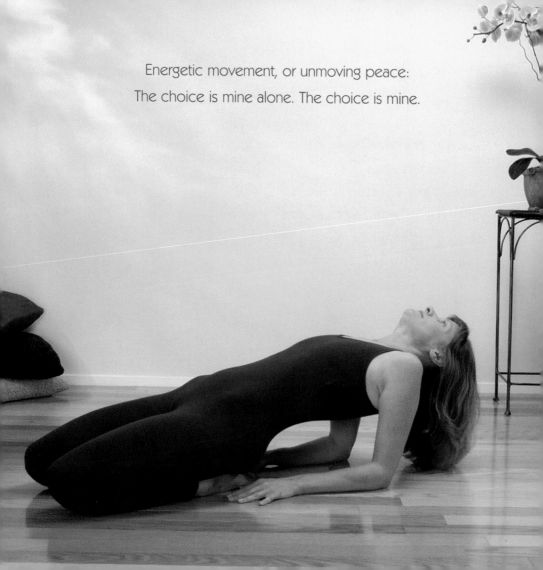

Energetic movement, or unmoving peace:
The choice is mine alone. The choice is mine.

*"Energetic movement, or unmoving
peace: The choice is mine alone.
The choice is mine."*

To exit, roll onto one side,
straighten your legs, and roll onto
your back. Bring your knees up,
wrap your arms around them, and
gently roll left and right a few
times to massage your lower back.
Then rest on your back.

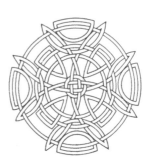

Variations

It is important to find a variation of this pose that enables you to be comfortable and relax completely. Think "deep, comfortable stretch" of the entire front side of the body. You may need one or more of the following variations to achieve comfort and relaxation:

If your neck tires, bring your chin to your chest (*figure a, page 117*) or rest the back of your head on a cushion . If needed, place a stack of blankets or cushions under your upper back, perhaps supporting your head as well (*figure b, page 117*); if your elbows do not reach the floor in this case, simply relax your arms at your sides.

If your ankles are uncomfortable, you can lessen the stretch by placing a rolled towel under the fronts of your ankles. If your knees are uncomfortable when flexed like this, you can decrease the flexion by placing a cushion between your ankles and buttocks (*figure c, page 117*). In this case, it is unlikely that you will be able to come down onto your elbows, so don't try. If your knees are still uncomfortable, do this pose on a chair.

If you are very flexible, you can get a deeper stretch by lowering all the way down onto the backs of your shoulders, arms resting at your sides. Do this, however, only if you can truly relax, avoid arching your lower back to the point of discomfort, and avoid separating your knees or lifting them off the floor.

You can also do this pose sitting sideways on a chair. Slide to one edge of the seat and place your feet under the chair, lowering your knees toward the floor. Bring your feet under the chair so the tops of your toes are on the floor (or as far as is comfortable.) Then lower yourself onto your elbows (*figure d*). Or use two chairs: sit on one as previously described, then lean back onto a stack of blankets or cushions placed on the other (*figure e*). Both these chair variations are useful for those with vulnerable knees. Finally, if your bed is firm enough to provide a reasonably solid foundation, you may be able to do these chair variations while sitting on the edge of the bed and leaning back onto the bed, instead of using the chair(s).

Cautions

Those with recent spinal injuries should do at most a gentle version of this pose, taking extra care to keep the pelvis tucked. Those with injured or vulnerable knees should do this pose on a chair.

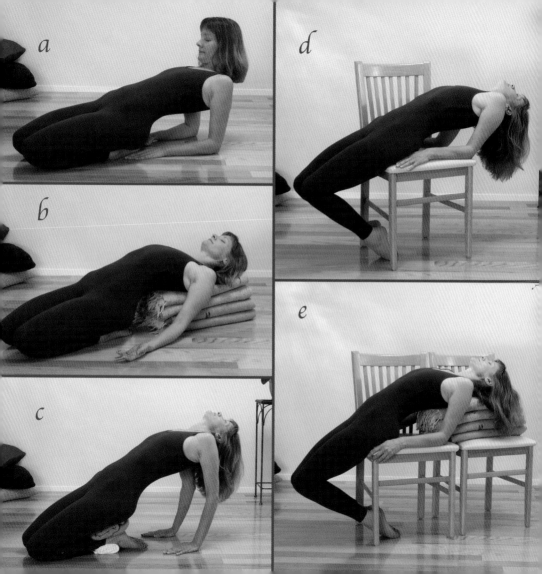

8. Posterior Stretching Pose

Sit upright with your legs straight in front of you, spine straight. Inhale as you bring your hands up the front of your body, stretching tall through your spine and arms. As you exhale, bend forward from your hips with a straight spine, and bring your hands down to the legs or floor, wherever they reach easily (*figure a*).

Continue in this "active phase" of the pose for several breaths as you inhale and lengthen the spine, then exhale and deepen the forward bend by bringing your navel toward your thighs. Keep your entire spine straight—including your neck—bending forward by relaxing the backs of your legs and buttocks rather than by rounding your spine. Relax your shoulders down away from your ears. Inhale and lengthen one last time, then exhale and release completely into the "relaxation phase" of the pose, allowing your spine and back muscles to soften (*figure b*).

From this point, go farther into the forward bend only through relaxation, not through effort. At all times, maintain a feeling of length and openness in the spine.

This pose helps release anxieties and fear, which often manifest as tension in the backs of the knees,

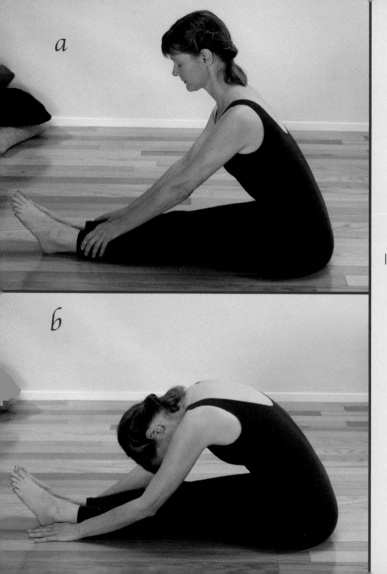

a

b

I am safe, I am sound.
All good things
come to me;
they give me peace.

buttocks, and lower back. Use Diaphragmatic Breathing as you hold the pose for up to 2 minutes, affirming,

> *"I am safe, I am sound.*
> *All good things come to me;*
> *they give me peace."*

To exit, on an inhalation, use your arms and abdominal and lower back muscles to straighten your spine once again, then lift your hands high overhead, drawing your torso to vertical and stretching your spine. Exhale and circle your hands out and down to your sides. Then lie on your back for at least 30 seconds, relaxing your spine and the entire back side of your body.

Variations

To maintain a straight spine in the active phase of the pose, you may need to sit on a cushion, with its front edge under your sit-bones to tilt your pelvis forward. If the cushion is thick, you may need another cushion under your knees to prevent hyperextension of the knee joints *(figure c)*.

If you are unable to achieve substantial relaxation and/or avoid hunching over in the pose, rest your arms and forehead on a chair seat *(figure d)*.

Cautions

If you have a weak lower back, engage the abdominal muscles

and back muscles to support it. Pregnant women and overweight persons should separate the feet enough to minimize pressure on the abdomen . Those with spinal injuries should stay in the active phase throughout, or if there is discomfort, do the Child Pose instead.

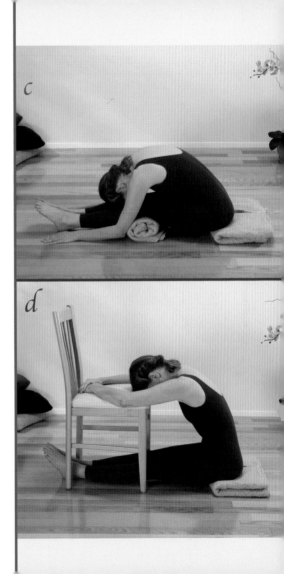

9. Fish Pose

Lie on your back and place your hands beneath your buttocks, wrists straight and palms down. Your elbows should be shoulder-width apart. As you inhale, press your sit-bones into your hands and elbows into the floor, slowly drawing your body up into a backward bend. Let your head slide closer to your body as you come up, but not so close that your neck bends backward sharply. Place very little weight on your head. Spread your shoulder blades wide.

Actively press your elbows into the floor, and sit-bones into the backs of your hands, in order to open the entire front of your torso and neck. This asana brings a feeling of ease and openness to your breathing and your mind. Visualize your breath—and your awareness—expanding in all directions, like ripples from a stone dropped into a pond. Hold the pose for 30 seconds, affirming,

"My soul floats on waves of cosmic light."

To exit, inhale and bring your chin to your chest, then exhale and slowly lower your back to the floor, starting with the lumbar spine and finishing with the head. Rest for 20–30 seconds, enjoying the sense of expansion.

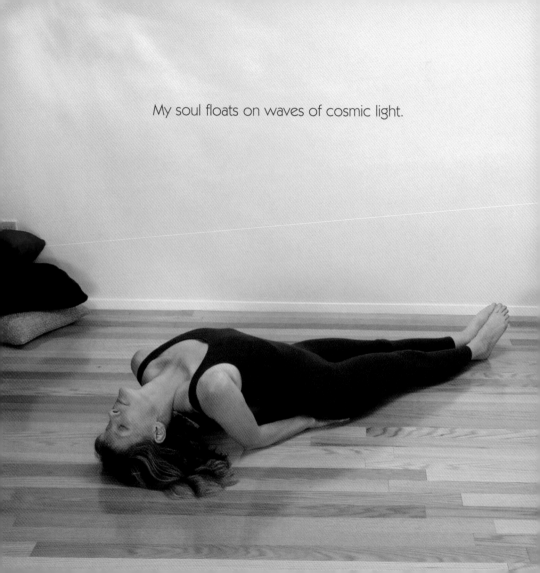

My soul floats on waves of cosmic light.

Cautions

Individuals with eye, ear, or sinus problems should keep the chin at the chest or rest the back of the head on a padded surface. Those with recent spinal injuries should avoid this pose.

✳ *10.*   Supine Twist

Lie on your back, arms at your sides. Bend your left knee and slide your left foot toward your buttocks. Shift your hips 4–6 inches to the left, then place your left foot on your right thigh, above the knee. Place your right hand on your left knee and stretch your left arm straight out to your side. Inhale and lengthen your spine, then exhale as you roll your lower body to the right, keeping your left shoulder on the floor and relaxing your left knee toward the floor. Lift your head slightly and rotate your gaze out over your outstretched left arm, then lower your head to the floor.

I open to the flow of God's
life within me.

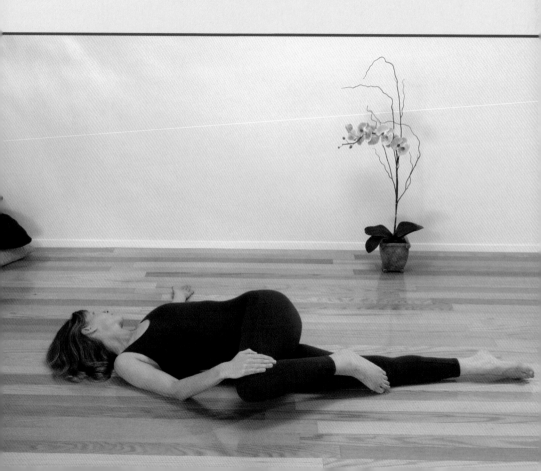

This pose releases tensions in the chest area, thereby opening the breath. It also stretches and relaxes the muscles along the spine, helping to open the "energy spine," the primary channel for subtle energy to flow in the body. (Like the physical spine, the energy spine extends from the tailbone up into the brain.) Hold the pose for at least 30 seconds, concentrating on letting go of tension and opening your spine so the energy can flow more freely. Affirm,

"I open to the flow of God's life within me."

To exit, rotate your head back to center, then inhale to lengthen your spine. As you exhale, roll your lower body back to center. Release your left foot to the floor, slide your hips back to center, straighten your left leg to the floor, and relax your arms to your sides. Rest for 10–15 seconds, enjoying the feeling of release around your spine before repeating the pose to the other side.

Variations

If your lower back is uncomfortable in the pose, bring your left knee closer to your right shoulder (vice versa when doing the other side of the pose).

If it's difficult to place the sole of your foot on the opposite thigh, above the knee, simply hook the toes behind the knee, with the ankle alongside the knee joint.

Pregnant women and overweight persons can bend the knee less to avoid abdominal compression.

Cautions

Those with hip replacements and recent spinal injuries should avoid this pose.

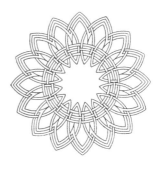

11.   Optional: The Calming Breath

This is a classical yoga technique for calming the mind. If you already feel able to go to sleep, omit this technique and go directly to 1:2 Breathing in Corpse Pose (#12 of this routine).

Sit upright on the edge of your bed, spine straight, left hand in your lap, and feet flat on the floor (or on a cushion if they do not reach the floor). Curl the first two fingers of your right hand to the palm, keeping the other fingers and thumb extended (figure a).

Bring the right thumb next to the right nostril, and the ring and little finger next to the left nostril. Use the Diaphragmatic Breath in this technique. Press the right nostril closed with the right thumb and inhale through the left nostril to a count of 6 (figure b). Then hold the breath to a count of 6 as you close the left nostril with the tips of the ring and little fingers of the right hand. Next lift the thumb off the right nostril and exhale through the right nostril to a count of 6. Immediately close the right nostril with the thumb, open the left, and inhale through the left nostril to a count of 6. Continue in this way, always inhaling through the left nostril and exhaling through the right nostril.

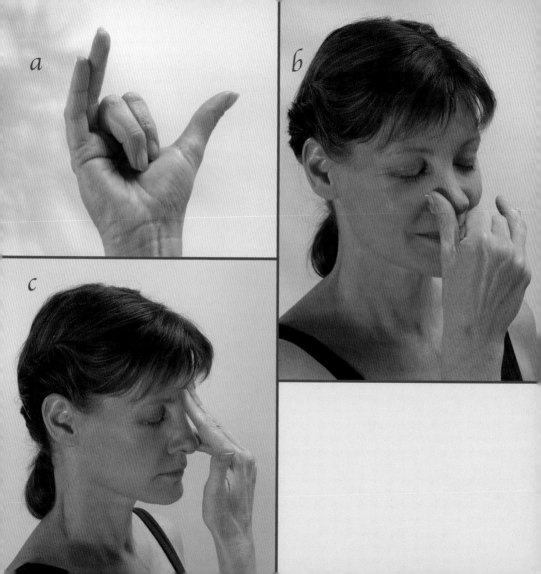

Do this technique with a sense of increasing calmness, until you feel ready to lie down and go to sleep.

(Note: The body's natural rhythms dictate that, at any given time, one or the other of your nostrils will be somewhat less open than the other. If this interferes with your practice of the Calming Breath, it is usually easy to open that nostril a bit more. If, for example, your right nostril is somewhat closed, lie on your left side and make a pillow for your head with your left arm. After a couple minutes in this position, breathing naturally, your right nostril should open up again. Then you can sit upright to practice the Calming Breath.)

Variations

If a 6-count is too long or too short, use whatever count works for you. In any case, *do not strain*.

For an even more relaxing technique, you can combine the Calming Breath with 1:2 Breathing (exhalations twice as long as the inhalations).

If the traditional right hand position described above is too uncomfortable, place the first two fingers of the right hand at the point between the eyebrows. Use the other fingers and thumb as described above *(figure c, page 129)*.

Caution

Pregnant women and persons with cardiovascular problems should hold the breath only briefly (2–4 counts).

✳ *12.* 1:2 Breathing in Corpse Pose
Turn off the lights and lie on your back in bed, with nothing left to do but go to sleep. Close your eyes. Stretch your legs away from your head to lengthen your spine. Slide your shoulders down away from your ears. Turn your inner arms and palms upward.

This is Corpse Pose. It promotes a deep feeling of peace and internal awareness. It is the ideal position for sleep (provided your pillow is not so thick that it causes your neck to be out of alignment with the rest of your spine).

Concentrate on your breathing, using Diaphragmatic Breathing. (If you still feel restless, you can begin with the Full Yogic Breath, then transition into Diaphragmatic Breathing.) Slowly lengthen your exhalations until they are twice as long as your inhalations. Measure the length of inhalations and exhalations by counting: if a 3-count inhalation feels best, gradually move toward 6-count exhalations. Or use a 2-count inhalation and 4-count exhalation, or 4 and 8 counts. All of these are 1:2 ratios between inhalation and exhalation; use whichever one is most comfortable and allows relaxed, even breathing. Longer counts are not the aim here; simply make your breathing as easy and natural as possible within this 1:2 ratio.

Do not force the 1:2 ratio right away; merely move in that direction. Do not control the breath any more than necessary; allow it to find its own 1:2 rhythm. If you find that the breath "wants" to pause after an inhalation or exhalation, let it do so without trying to prolong or shorten the pause. Continue the 1:2 ratio until you go to sleep. (If the breath evolves from a Full Yogic Breath to a Diaphragmatic Breath, that's fine.)

During relaxed sleep, you naturally breathe diaphragmatically with a 1:2 ratio (approximately). By breathing diaphragmatically with this ratio *before* sleep, you are placing body and mind "in sync" with a relaxed state of sleep. Unwavering concentration on the breath is the key. Whenever your mind strays from observing the breath, bring it back. You may also find it helpful to turn the eyes downward behind closed eyelids, for that is their usual position during sleep.

Variation

Yogis say that it's ideal to sleep on your back. If you prefer to sleep on your side, practice a few minutes of 1:2 Breathing on your back, then turn onto your side for more 1:2 Breathing. (One knee should be atop the other, side by side; otherwise, your spine will tend to twist.) If the 1:2 ratio is difficult while lying on your side, simply make the exhalation as long as is comfortable. Do not, in any case, sleep on your belly; that position makes it more difficult to breathe and is unhealthy for your spine.

Additional "into Sleep" Techniques

You may also find that one or more of the following optional techniques will help take you into sleep. You can use them after—or instead of—1:2 Breathing in Corpse Pose. These techniques and 1:2 Breathing are also helpful if you wake up during the night and have trouble going back to sleep. (*See Chapter Eight.*)

It's usually best to choose just one of these and practice it, but once you are comfortable with these techniques (including 1:2 Breathing in Corpse Pose) individually, you might wish to combine two or more of them. As long as the combination feels natural, this approach can help you engage more fully in the gentle journey into sleep. Remember, however, that we offer you these options to facilitate your "into sleep" experience, not to complicate it. So whatever you do, keep it simple, natural, and relaxing.

All of these techniques are done while lying on your back in bed, eyes closed, ready for sleep. The choice is yours and will depend on your own state of mind and personal preferences.

20-Part Progressive Relaxation

This technique is a more relaxing variant of 20-Part Body Recharging. Slowly move up the body, consciously relaxing each of the twenty body parts shown in the accompanying drawing, one by one. As you inhale, focus your attention completely on that body part. Hold the breath for 1–2 counts, and as you exhale, relax that part completely. Feel that, in relaxation, you are also withdrawing all your awareness from that body part. If you find it helpful, lightly tense the body part as you hold your breath, then relax it as you exhale.

One "pass" through the body consists of focusing on the twenty body parts in the order indicated in the drawing. You may wish to dwell a bit longer on body parts in which you chronically hold tension—e.g., abdomen or neck—doing the exercise two or more times before moving to the next part. If you are holding tension in any

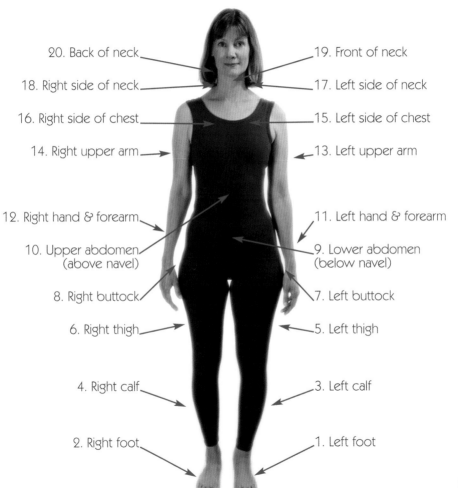

20. Back of neck

19. Front of neck

18. Right side of neck

17. Left side of neck

16. Right side of chest

15. Left side of chest

14. Right upper arm

13. Left upper arm

12. Right hand & forearm

11. Left hand & forearm

10. Upper abdomen (above navel)

9. Lower abdomen (below navel)

8. Right buttock

7. Left buttock

6. Right thigh

5. Left thigh

4. Right calf

3. Left calf

2. Right foot

1. Left foot

135

body parts other than these twenty, add those parts to the sequence.

Do as many passes as you find helpful, allowing (but not forcing) longer and longer pauses between the breaths on each pass. If you choose the light tension option, use it only on the first pass.

You can use 20-Part Progressive Relaxation before, after, or along with 1:2 Breathing. If you use light tension, then it's best to do 20-Part Progressive Relaxation before or along with 1:2 Breathing.

Visualization with Breath Control

Lie still and mentally observe the breath—not controlling it, just allowing its steady rhythm to soothe you, like ocean waves gently stroking the shore on a calm day. After a time, inhale deeply, then exhale slowly and completely, as if with a sigh; feel that you are surrendering yourself to an infinity of peace. Hold the breath out as long as you can comfortably, and affirm mentally, "Peace, peace, peace." Visualize an ocean of peace spreading out in all directions around you. Or think of peace as gathering protectively around you in great, soft clouds. Or use any other visual image that helps you feel more peaceful, more secure. Inhale when you need to do so. You might find it soothing to rest one or both hands on the belly.

Repeat this breathing and visualization process 6–12 times (in concert with 1:2 Breathing if you like). If you are still awake after that, continue calmly watching the breath, without controlling it or letting your mind wander. Let the breath lead you into sleep.

Withdrawal from Outward Awareness

In yoga, there are two common approaches to dealing with distractions. One is to concentrate on the distraction, so that your deepening concentration will eventually take you beyond the distraction. In the case of insomnia, breathing can sometimes distract you from sleep (the sound of it, for example, or lack of ease in breathing). The approach taken in 1:2 Breathing is to focus on that distraction.

The second approach is to withdraw your attention from the distraction and place it on something else. That is our approach in this technique: withdraw your attention from the breath and all other distractions. After all, when you are asleep, you are unaware of your breath, body, or senses. Therefore it makes sense to prepare for sleep by withdrawing your attention from all of these.

Here's how:

Inhale and tense the entire body, then throw the breath out, relaxing the body completely. Do this several times. Then forget your breath (even though it will still be flowing). Be indifferent to any sounds the body may make, such as your breathing or heartbeat, or any other bodily sensations or environmental noises. Don't try to push the sensations away; simply ignore them.

Be equally indifferent to any thoughts that arise in your mind. If thoughts come—and they will—it's okay; just don't get involved with them. Simply let them pass by like clouds on a breezy day.

Where *should* you place your attention? Imagine how you would feel after a week without sleep: you would feel so sleepy that you could sleep anywhere. Concentrate on that feeling. Absorb your mind in it. If you can give all your attention to that feeling, making it your foremost reality, it will carry you into sleep.

Note: Do not combine this technique with any of the other "into sleep" techniques, but you could practice it *after* one of the others if you wish.

Affirmation

In addition to their use with asanas to calm and focus out-of-control thoughts and energy, affirmations can help you take the next step: going directly into sleep. Done properly, they will help you internalize and focus the mind, rise above a restless mind or agitated emotions, and relax into sleep.

As with asana affirmations, for best results it is important to *feel* the state of consciousness that the affirmation suggests. For example, suppose you are unable to sleep because of anxiety over an important meeting tomorrow. First, choose an affirmation to fit this situation, such as "I relax and cast aside all mental burdens." Repeat it with a feeling of increasing freedom from concern over the meeting. Imagine that freedom, feel it, enjoy it. (Don't allow yourself to feel guilty about sleeping, by the way. You've already decided not to stay up and prepare more for the meeting. So go to sleep!) Gradually move from silent repetition of the affirmation into a wordless absorption in that happy freedom and the relaxation that it brings. Know that the freedom and relaxation will help you sleep better, and thus have a more successful meeting tomorrow.

As you affirm, let your breath be smooth and natural, not controlling it at all. Or if you like, combine the affirmation with 1:2 breathing. For example:

Inhaling (3 counts): *"I relax and ..."*

Exhaling (6 counts): *"... cast aside all mental burdens."*

Choosing an Affirmation

You might wish to use one of your favorite asana affirmations to take you into sleep. Or it might help you to use an affirmation that addresses a particular sleep-impairing state of mind (see page 141). Or you might wish to create your own affirmation, as we'll discuss shortly. In any case, as you silently repeat the affirmation, the key to success is to absorb yourself more and more deeply in the essential feeling of the affirmation, until the words melt away into that feeling.

Some of these affirmations were developed or inspired by highly advanced yoga practitioners (see footnotes). If one resonates with you, try it. If you wish to modify one, please see the guidelines following.

As another option, many people find that a favorite spiritual quotation, used as an affirmation, helps them relax into sleep. Choices could include a Bible quotation (e.g., the 23rd Psalm, the Lord's Prayer), verses from the Bhagavad Gita, the Prayer of St. Francis ("Lord, make me an instrument of Thy peace. ..."), or a quotation from a favorite saint. Again, try to go beyond mechanical repetition; melt into the feeling of what you are affirming.

To Counter...	Affirmation
General inability to sleep	◆ With every breath, I relax toward deep, peaceful sleep.
	◆ Through slowly drifting waters, I sink into stillness.
	◆ I soften into the soothing blanket of sleep.
	◆ I open my mind to the gentle caress of sleep.
Preoccupation with problems, people, projects, etc.	◆ I relax and cast aside all mental burdens.[1]
	◆ I relax from outer involvement into my inner haven of peace.[2]
Worry, insecurity, fear	◆ I am safe, I am sound. All good things come to me; they give me peace.[2]
	◆ I relax in perfect faith that what I need will come to me.
Jealousy	◆ I rejoice in the good fortune of all; thus do I find freedom. [3]
Anger, resentment, hurt	◆ The warmth of my forgiveness melts away all pain.
	◆ I radiate love to all, for loving heals my heart.
	◆ Thy truth lives within me, not in the opinions of others.[3]
Unhappiness over circumstances	◆ I am grateful for the goodness in my life.
	◆ All that happens is for the good; it is a gift from Thee.
	◆ This too shall pass.
Illness, injury, or pain	◆ Every breath fills me with healing and wholeness.
	◆ Thy healing light permeates every fiber of my being. [4]
	◆ I am well, for perfection is in me.[4]

1 *Praecepta Lessons*, by Paramhansa Yogananda, 1938. Currently available in *Scientific Healing Affirmations*, by Paramhansa Yogananda, Self-Realization Fellowship.

2 *The Art and Science of Raja Yoga*, by Swami Kriyananda.

3 *Affirmations for Self-Healing*, by J. Donald Walters (Swami Kriyananda).

4 *Metaphysical Meditations*, by Paramhansa Yogananda, 1932 edition, Self-Realization Fellowship

Guidelines for Creating Your Own Affirmations

If you would like to develop your own affirmation or modify an existing one, the following guidelines will help you make it more effective:

* If you can identify a specific mental or emotional obstacle to sleep (e.g., worry or grief), tailor your affirmation to address that obstacle.

* Usually, an affirmation is a *positive* statement. A negative statement such as "I am never restless or agitated" could lead your subconscious mind (which tends to be very literal) to focus on "restless and agitated" instead of "never." The effect could be the opposite of what you seek.

* Be realistic. For example, it may not be realistic to affirm, "I will be asleep in one minute." In fact, using any time limit could make you feel pressured and thus push you away from sleep rather than toward it.

* Affirm in the present tense, usually. The future tense ("will") can rob your affirmation of definiteness and immediacy. For example, "I relax into deep, peaceful sleep" is preferable to "I will relax into deep, peaceful

sleep." (Note: in some affirmations, however, "will" works perfectly well.)

• Use language that appeals to your feeling nature, not just your intellect. Thus will you more easily become absorbed in a sleep-friendly state. For example, as you affirm, "I am safe, I am sound. All good things come to me; they give me peace," feel what it's like to be secure and cared for; feel the contentment of knowing that a continuous stream of beneficial people, events, and circumstances is coming your way. This will help you be more relaxed and receptive to sleep. (Note: Visual images or pleasant sensations of any kind are helpful in engaging your feeling nature. Some of the above affirmations are excellent examples of how to bring imagery into affirmations.)

• Affirmations can be of any length. Short affirmations require less conscious effort and may help you stay focused. Longer ones also can be effective, perhaps by conveying a more vivid image, but make sure that they do not over-engage your intellect or make memorization too difficult.

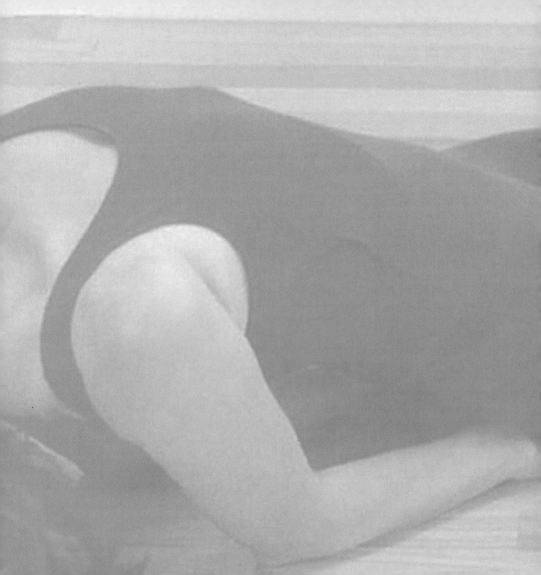

✸

Chapter Eight

When You Wake Up During the Night

Unfortunately, insomnia isn't only about being unable to fall sleep at bedtime. There may be nights when you are able to get to sleep, but wake up in the middle of the night and are unable to get back to sleep. There are two possible strategies in this case, depending on whether or not sleep feels close at hand.

Almost Asleep

First, you may feel as though you are still close to sleep, and you require just "a little something" to put you over the edge of wakefulness and return to sleep. In this case, stay in bed and practice 1:2 Breathing in Corpse Pose and/or any of the Additional "into Sleep" Techniques described in Chapter Seven:

- 20-Part Progressive Relaxation (one or more passes, with longer and longer pauses between the breaths on each pass—with or without light tension on the first pass)—page 134

- Visualization with Breath Control (6–12 times)—page 136

- Withdrawal from Outward Awareness—page 137

- Affirmation (as desired, with or without breath control) —page 138

Wide Awake … for Now

On the other hand, what if you wake up in the middle of the night and are wide awake? Your mind may begin to race, or bodily tensions or agitation may creep in—or both may happen. In this case, you might as well concede that sleep is not "just around the corner," and that you need to do something a bit more active in order to get back to sleep.

One option is to get up and do something relaxing, such as reading, until you feel sleepy once again, then follow the "Almost Asleep" approach above. (Just a note about reading: Some books are written to be "page-turners," the type of book you just can't put down. Obviously, these will not help you fall asleep. Choose something that is a bit more calming—perhaps even boring!)

Alternatively, you can try the following approach.

Release Any Bodily Tensions

First, look for any bodily tensions that may be keeping you awake. For example, there might be "anxiety knots" in your stomach, or emotional pain around your heart, or even bodily aches or muscle tensions with no apparent connection to mental states. Often such tensions can be relieved simply by staying in bed and tensing and relaxing that area of the body several times to take control of the tension and release it (as in 20-Part Body Recharging).

If that's not sufficient, then get out of bed and do any of the exercises in this book that address that area of the body. As you consciously relax those body parts, feel yourself becoming calmer and more at rest.

For example, if your legs become restless in response to thoughts of "getting into gear" and doing something, you could relax them by doing the Posterior Stretching Pose. For emotional upset or neck and shoulder tension, you could try the Hare Pose, using the Full Yogic Breath to help you assert control over your body.

In any case, don't do many exercises unless that feels appropriate; just focus on the immediate need so you can return to sleep as soon as possible. Once you have relieved the tensions, get into bed and practice 1:2 Breathing in Corpse Pose for a time. Often that will take you back into sleep, but if not, then continue with any of the Additional "into Sleep" Techniques (*see Chapter Seven*) that you think will be helpful.

Dealing with Mental Wakefulness

Finally, suppose there's no apparent physical involvement—or you've already eliminated it as above. Your body feels relaxed and ready for sleep, but your mind is still wide awake and churning.

In this case, keep your body relaxed as you work primarily with breathing techniques. Sit upright and do a few Full Yogic Breaths to grab your mind's attention. Then shift into the Calming Breath until your mind feels calm and relaxed. Then lie down and do 1:2 Breathing in Corpse Pose.

As always with breathing techniques, concentrate one-pointedly on the breath. Don't allow your mind to drift, don't worry about your problems (especially the insomnia problem!), and don't wonder about your performance of a technique. Just place your full attention on your breath. If needed, you can also employ any of the Additional "into Sleep" Techniques *(see Chapter Seven)*. Remember: the more deeply you absorb yourself in the practice of any technique, the more effective it becomes.

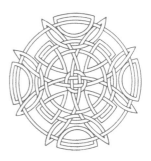

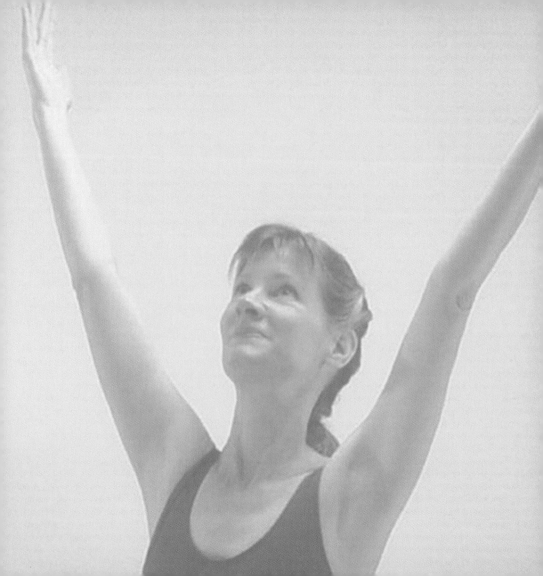

✳

Chapter Nine

Secrets of a Great Night's Sleep

Cooperating with Your Body Clock

Your "body clock," as we've mentioned, is a real key to deep, sound sleep. You can enlist its aid, rather than fighting it, by following some simple steps. Just as your body can learn bad sleep habits, it can also learn good ones.

First, choose a bedtime and awakening time that fits your lifestyle and temperament. Make sure you're realistically allowing yourself enough hours of sleep, since this will become your daily routine. As much as possible, stay with the same hours of sleep each night. Within two weeks, your body clock will be aligned with your new sleep and awakening times. Particularly in the beginning, you should follow the same sleep time routine even on days off from your normal responsibilities. Having a regular awakening time is particularly key in setting your body's clock, and you should get up then no matter how poorly you've slept. It's best not to take naps during the day even if you are sleepy. You'll find that you'll be less ready for sleep at bedtime if you do.

Since your body keys on a decline in your body temperature for starting sleep, avoid hot baths or vigorous exercise within three hours of your bedtime. We do recommend regular exercise, but try to get it earlier in the day. Also, you'll want to have your bedroom cool at bedtime.

To take advantage of your brain's own sleep-inducing chemical, melatonin, get some bright light exposure each day soon after awakening. This will decrease your brain's melatonin levels early in the day. With less melatonin you'll be more awake and alert. We recommend 30-45 minutes worth of light exposure as early in the day as possible. If sunlight isn't available because you wake up when it's still dark, bright artificial light may be the best you can do. In the evening, as you approach bedtime, keep the room lights low so your melatonin levels will increase to help ready you for sleep.

Making Sure Your Body Will Be Ready for Deep, Natural Sleep

You should avoid any stimulating drugs, including caffeine and nicotine, within six hours of bedtime. If you must take a prescription drug for medical reasons, such as a stimulating asthma inhaler, use it as far away from bedtime as possible. You might consider asking your physician if you can change the timing or dose of any medication that is affecting your sleep. If you are a women awakened by hot flashes, you may want to discuss hormone replacement therapy with your doctor. Women with hot flashes who can't or don't want to take hormones may get relief from hot flashes by using the drug Effexor, a common antidepressant. If pain is awakening you, try taking a bedtime dose of a mild pain reliever—just make sure it doesn't contain caffeine. We also suggest that you not use any alcohol or other recreational drugs within six hours of bedtime because these may cause disturbed sleep patterns. It's best for sleep if you don't use them at all. Both marijuana and alcohol, for example, can predispose you to anxiety or depression, which in turn may result in a sleep problem.

A bedtime snack can be very beneficial in helping you get to sleep and not be bothered with feeling hungry during the night. Bananas or warm milk are both good choices since they are high in the amino acid tryptophan that can help induce sleep. In the yoga tradition, starchy carbohydrates and sweets are considered poor choices for a bedtime snack. You can choose a light snack you enjoy. Just be sure it is not spicy and does not cause heartburn. You should experiment with what works well for you.

Having a regular exercise program is one of the most important aids to good sleep. Including thirty minutes of exercise at least five times a week will work wonders for your sleep, and will help you feel more vigorous during the day. Brisk walking is fine, but exercising harder is better, if you are fit. You can split your thirty minutes of exercise into smaller segments and spread them over the day if that works better for you.

You should limit your fluid intake as you get close to bedtime so you won't be awakened by a need to go to the bathroom.

Make Your Bedroom Perfect for Sleeping

Your bedroom should be as dark and as quiet as possible. If you have problems with noise from outside (or a snoring sleep partner) awakening you, consider getting a "sound generator." It can make a quiet nature sound, such as a burbling brook or waves on a beach, or it can just be static "white noise." Any of these will mask other sounds so they don't disturb you as you sleep. You can also achieve a good masking sound by simply setting a radio so that it produces a bland static sound. You can even wear earplugs, but we don't recommend this as a regular practice since it can irritate your ear canals.

Make your bed as comfortable as possible. Your sheets, pillow, mattress, and blankets should all feel pleasant to the touch and be the right weight and firmness for you. You can improve the softness of your current bed inexpensively by adding a foam pad or air pad on top of your regular mattress. If you have trouble with heavy blankets but like to stay warm at night, consider a down or fiberfill comforter instead.

You bedroom should be as cool as is comfortable for you. Remember your body's temperature needs to fall in order for you go to sleep, so you don't want to get overheated. Be sure not to have so many blankets on at night that you sweat, a sign you are too hot for sound sleep.

Your bed (and bedroom if possible) should be reserved for only sleep and sex. You want always to have the association in your mind when you see your bed, "this bed is where I sleep soundly!" If you want to watch TV, read, pay bills, work at your computer, chat with your spouse, or use the telephone, it's best to do that in another room or at least sitting up in a chair. Wait to head for bed until you feel a little sleepy at bedtime.

If you don't fall asleep in 20-30 minutes get up and go read until you feel sleepy again. If you awaken in the night and are awake for more than ten minutes, get up and do something else quiet until you feel sleepy.

It's fine to set an alarm clock if you might not wake up on your own, but face the clock away from you so that you can't "watch the clock" if you awaken at night.

In the yoga tradition, it is also recommended that the head of your bed point in any direction but west.

It's Close to Bedtime

This is a perfect time to do your Ananda Yoga postures, and we suggest that you do our routine just before you get into bed since this will relax you mentally and physically for sleep. You should emphasize quiet and relaxation in your thoughts and movements as you prepare for sleep. This would also be a nice time to say some prayers for your loved ones and yourself, and meditate for a while if you know how.

If you need to take a sleep medication, take it about one hour before sleep so its effect is maximum as you head for bed. If you are taking valerian as a sleep-inducing agent instead of a prescription medication, this would be the time to take it. We don't recommend melatonin tablets.

It's good to avoid television or computer use close to bedtime since they are bright light sources that encourage your body to be alert and they often keep your mind engaged with thoughts that will interfere with sleep. Try turning off the TV or computer at least an hour before bed.

Take Advantage of These Affirmations

In Chapters Six and Seven, we offered a variety of techniques that can help you make the "last leg" of your journey into sleep. Although affirmation is just one of those techniques, we strongly recommend that you learn how to use it, because taking you into sleep is just one of its benefits. As we've mentioned, it is also an excellent way of retraining your mind and making it an ongoing ally in your quest for deep sleep. Affirmations are particularly effective when used as you fall asleep and just as you awaken. At those times, you actually have special access to your subconscious mind, so the affirmations can be even more effective than usual. When the positive feeling of an affirmation is your last thought as you drift off, you will find that it deepens your sleep. Also, your bedtime affirmation will be another habit you will associate with going to sleep, and within weeks, just saying that in your mind will make you drowsy!

On awakening, we suggest you say to yourself, "I am awake, energetic, enthusiastic!" You can also say this while doing some gentle stretches after you are out of bed. It's an excellent way to train your mind that it is time to be wide-awake. We also recommend doing the 20-Part Body Recharging exercise (see Chapter Seven) upon awakening, to make sure your body and brain are wide awake and energized for the day; if you like, you can even do it while lying in bed before rising.

What to Do If You Are Still Having Trouble

While we expect that our program will work well for almost everybody, if you are still having insomnia trouble after one month, you may benefit from a visit to your physician. You can take this book along to show him you are practicing excellent sleep habits and daytime routines. If you need to take medication for a short time, we suggest Ambien or Sonata as first choice, with generic temazepam as an inexpensive alternative. For medication therapy for more than a month, for women, we suggest a trial of the non-addictive anti-depressant trazadone (Deseryl) starting with low doses and increasing very slowly. Since men may have side effects to trazadone (Deseryl), we recommend mirtazapine (Remeron), starting with the lowest effective dose. For really difficult cases, a visit to a sleep specialist may help.

If, after reading this book, you suspect you have an underlying physical problem affecting your sleep such as asthma or sleep apnea, do discuss this with your physician early on. You can still do the program outlined in this book safely, and it will be beneficial. If you think that anxiety or depression may be a factor in your insomnia, we also suggest you get this evaluated by your physician, along with using our system.

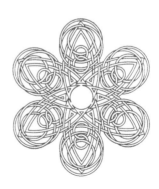

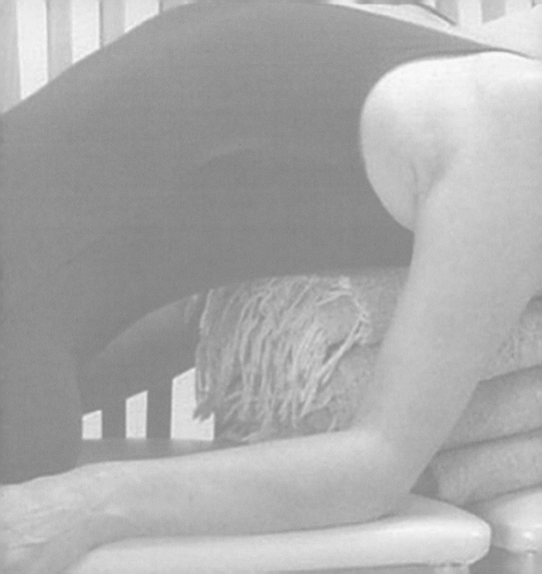

✴

Chapter Ten

Putting It All Together

This last section is a simple check-list you can use you to determine your new sleep schedule and to be sure that you are following all our guidelines. You may want to look at this list every evening for the first two weeks you are doing this program to refine your answers and to see that you are remembering everything.

Sleep Times

How many hours do I sleep on nights when I awaken refreshed (estimate the average amount to within a half an hour)? _____

To get in the number of hours of sleep I calculated in the last question, what time will I need to go to bed? _____
Awaken?_____

Am I doing well at getting up every morning at my wake-up time even if I haven't slept well? _____(hint: The answer should be yes!)

(Remember, you should try to use the same bedtime and awakening time every night for at least the first two weeks and as often as possible after that.)

Getting Your Bedroom Ready

Is my bed comfortable and inviting? _____

Is there anything I can do to improve my sleeping comfort? _____

Is my bedroom dark and quiet enough? _____

Do I need to use sound masking if it's noisy (or my bed partner snores)?

Is the bedroom's temperature cool enough for sleep? _____

Do I have the clock positioned so I can't see it at night? _____

Have I transferred all the TV, computer, and all activities except sleep and sex away from my bed? _____

Daytime Habits

Have I established an exercise routine? _____

What kind of exercise? _____ How often? _____

Am I getting sunlight exposure first thing in the morning (or bright artificial light?)_____How long? _____

Am I limiting my caffeine intake and use of other stimulants like cigarettes? _____

If not, am I at least trying to keep their use six hours away from bedtime? _____

Am I keeping alcohol and other recreational drugs at least six hours away from bedtime? _____

Have I spoken with my physician about any medication that may be hurting my sleep? _____

Am I limiting my fluid intake close to bedtime (so I won't need to urinate at night)? _____

Am I limiting my TV and computer use so that they end at least an hour before bed? _____

It's Time for Bed

Am I waiting until I'm sleepy before I go to bed? _____

Am I ready to do my Ananda Yoga postures nightly to help prepare my body and mind for sleep? _____

Am I doing my postures slowly and restfully to get myself ready for sleep? _____

Have I taken on schedule any medication for sleep that's been prescribed? _____

Do I have my "going to sleep" and "awakening" affirmations clear in my mind, and am I ready to do them? _____

If I'm not asleep in twenty minutes, do I get out of bed until I felt sleepy again? _____

If I awaken in the night and am not back to sleep in ten minutes, do I get up and read until I felt sleepy again? _____

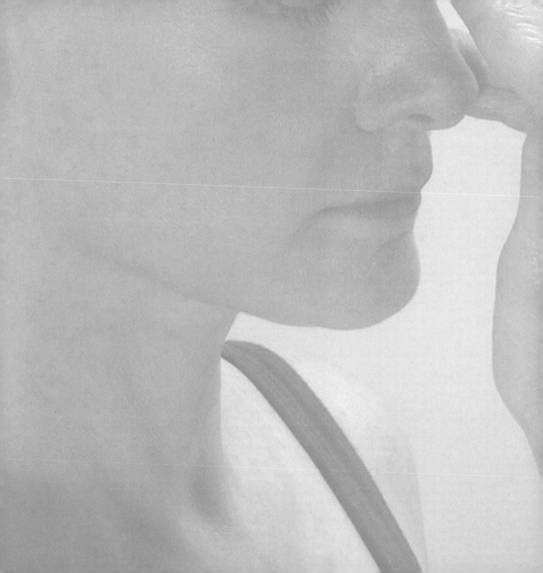

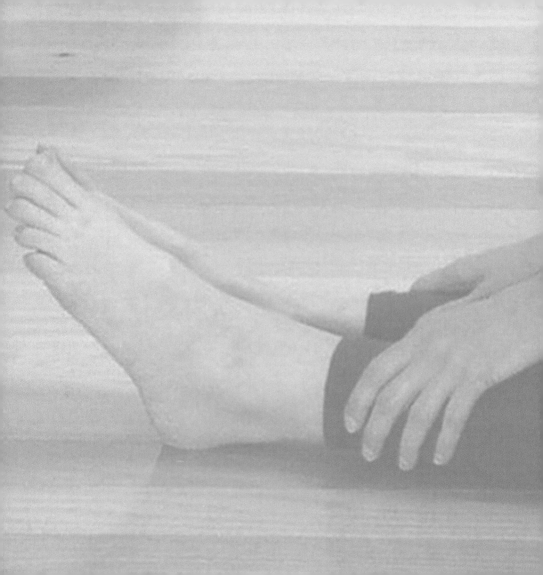

✺

Chapter Eleven

Next Steps with Ananda Yoga

You will find additional information on Ananda Yoga and Ananda Yoga Therapy on the web at www.AnandaYoga.org.

We hope that at some point you will begin practicing a more general Ananda Yoga routine. In addition to helping prevent and relieve insomnia, this will bring your entire body and mind into greater harmony. You can increase the benefits of the postures even more by adding the practice of meditation, the most powerful technique in all of yoga.

To help you move in these directions, we recommend the resources below. The books and videos can be found at many bookstores; most are also available through Crystal Clarity Publishers (800.424.1055/530.478.7600 or www.crystalclarity.com).

The Expanding Light retreat is the primary teaching center for Ananda Yoga and Ananda Sangha, the worldwide spiritual work of which Ananda Yoga is a part. Located in the beautiful Sierra Nevada foothills of Northern California, the retreat is open year-round and offers programs in Ananda Yoga, Ananda Yoga Therapy, meditation, meditation therapy, health and healing, yoga and meditation teacher certification, personalized retreats, and much more. Private sessions of Ananda Yoga and Ananda Yoga Therapy are also available.

For a free brochure, call 800-346-5350 or 530-478-7518, e-mail info@expandinglight.org, or visit www.expandinglight.org.

You can also receive training at various Ananda teaching centers throughout the U.S. and Europe. In addition, Ananda teachers travel widely, giving lectures and workshops. Visit www.ananda.org for more information.

Books

Ananda Yoga for Higher Awareness, *by Swami Kriyananda.* This is the definitive book on Ananda Yoga, by its founder. In addition to teaching a wide range of yoga postures, it offers breathing exercises and sample routines.

Yoga Therapy for Headache Relief, *by Peter Van Houten, M.D., and Gyandev Rich McCord, Ph.D.* Its format is similar to this book specifically for treating headaches..

The Art and Science of Raja Yoga, *by Swami Kriyananda.* This book/CD set includes everything in Ananda Yoga for Higher Awareness, plus many of the main aspects of the broader science of yoga, including philosophy, meditation, diet, and health.

How to Meditate, *by John Jyotish Novak.* This book outlines the basics of meditation, including a classical yoga meditation technique.

Meditation for Starters, *by Swami Kriyananda.* This book/CD combination is an introduction to meditation; the CD includes a guided meditation practice.

Affirmations for Self-Healing, *by J. Donald Walters (Swami Kriyananda).* This book offers affirmations and prayers for developing specific character qualities within yourself.

Books by Other Publishers

Metaphysical Meditations, *by Paramhansa Yogananda,* Self-

Realization Fellowship Publishers. This book offers affirmations and prayers for a wide variety of purposes, from psychological to spiritual.

Scientific Healing Affirmations, 1924 Edition, by Paramhansa Yogananda, Self-Realization Fellowship Publishers. This book offers affirmations and prayers for a wide variety of purposes, from physical to psychological to spiritual.

Videos

Yoga for Busy People, by Gyandev Rich McCord and Lisa Powers. This video offers three 25-minute Ananda Yoga routines, one each for developing vitality, calmness, and harmonizing the heart.

Yoga for Emotional Healing, by Lisa Powers. This video describes the basics of the Ananda Yoga approach to working with emotions, then offers a 45-minute practice routine.

Yoga to Awaken the Chakras, by Gyandev McCord. This video describes the workings of the chakras (subtle energy centers within you), and how to use Ananda Yoga to work with the chakras to raise your consciousness, using a 45-minute practice routine.

Meditation Therapy for Stress and Change, *by Jyotish Novak.* How to use meditation practices for dealing with the inevitable stresses and changes that life brings.

Meditation Therapy for Health and Healing, *by Jyotish Novak.* How to use meditation practices for maintaining and restoring health, vitality, and harmony on many levels.

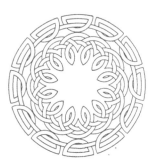

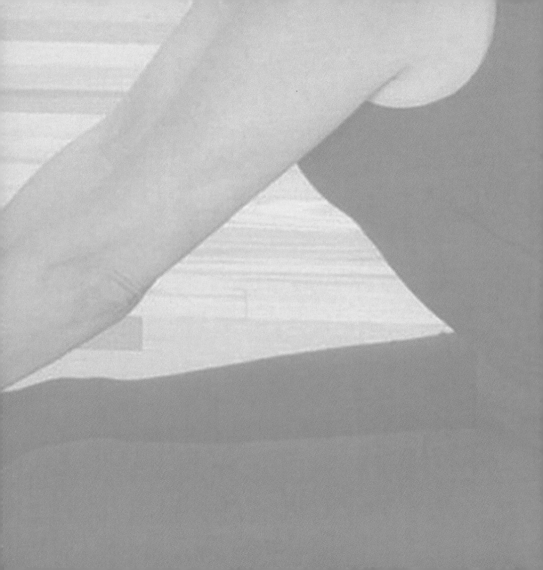

Medical Bibliography

Ancoli-Israel, Sonia (1994). Sleep Disorders, Lecture for Post Graduate Physicians, San Diego, California.

Boivin, D.B. et al. (1996). Dose-Response Relationships for Resetting of Human Circadian Clock by Light. *Nature*, 379:540-542.

Dinges, David F. (2000). Sleep, Sleep Deprivation, and Affect. Lecture at 6th Annual Wisconsin Symposium on Emotion.

Grantcharov, T. et al. (2002). Laparoscopic Performance After One Night On Call in a Surgical Department: Prospective Study. *British Medical Journal USA*, Volume 2, January 2002.

Guilleminault, C. et al. (1995). Nondrug Treatment Trials in Psychophysiologic Insomnia, *Archives Internal Medicine*, 155:838-84.

Hypnotic Drugs (2000), *The Medical Letter*, Volume 42, Issue 1084.

Jacobs, Gregg. (1998). Say Goodnight to Insomnia. Owl Books.

Karni, A. et al. (1994). Dependence on REM Sleep of Overnight Improvement of a Perceptual Skill, *Science*, 265:679-682.

Lapuma, John. (2002). Clinical Briefs: Melatonin for Jet Lag, Alternative Medicine Alert, November 1, 2002 issue.

Marcolina, Susan. (2002). Valerian Root for Insomnia. *Alternative Medicine Alert*, 5:77-80.

Morin, C.M. et al. (1999). Behavioral and Pharmacological Therapies for Late-Life Insomnia: A Randomized Controlled Trial, *JAMA*, 281:991-999.

Morriss, R. et al. (1993). Abnormalities of Sleep in Patients with the Chronic Fatigue Syndrome, *British Medical Journal*, 306:1161-1164.

Radecki, S.E. and Brunton, S.A. (1993). Management of Insomnia in Office-Based Practice: National Prevalence and Therapeutic Patterns. *Archives Family Medicine*, 2:1129-1134.

Robbins, J. and Gottleib, F. (1990). Sleep Deprivation and Cognitive Testing in Internal Medicine House Staff. *Western Journal of Medicine*, 152:82-86.

Rumble, R. and Morgan, K. (1992). Hypnotics, Sleep, and Mortality in Elderly People, *Journal of the American Geriatric Society*, 40:787-791.

Sleep Disorders, a four-article symposium, Postgraduate Medicine, Volume 107, Number 3, March 2000: Mahowald, M. Introduction to Series; Mahowald, M. What is Causing Excessive Daytime Sleepiness; Attarian, H. Helping Patients Who Say They Cannot Sleep; Mahowald, M. Parasomnias.

Solowij, N. et al. (2002). Cognitive Functioning of Long-Term Heavy Cannabis Users Seeking Treatment. *JAMA*, 287:1123-31.

Weilburg, Jeffrey (2000). Approach to the Patient with Insomnia. *Primary Care Medicine: Office Evaluation and Management of the Adult Patient*, Fourth Edition, Lippincott, Williams, and Wilkins.

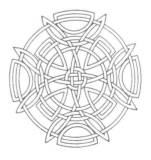